Detoxification and Healing: The Way to Perfect Health

Dr. Susan's Healthy Living
drsusanshealthyliving.com

Facebook.com/DrSusanRichards
drsusanshealthyliving@gmail.com
(650) 561-9978

I0417243

Mention of specific companies or products in this book does not suggest endorsement by the author or publisher. Internet addresses and telephone numbers for resources provided in this book were accurate at the time it went to press.

ISBN 978-1511943635

Note

The information in this book is meant to complement the advice and guidance of your physician, not replace it. It is very important that any person who has medical problems be evaluated by a physician. If you are under the care of a physician, you should discuss any major changes in your regimen with him or her. Because this is a book and not a medical consultation, keep in mind that the information presented here may not apply in your particular case. In view of individual medical requirements, new research, and government regulations, it is the responsibility of the reader to validate health practices and treatments with a physician or health service.

Table of Contents

Part I: How Detoxification Benefits Peak Performance and Health................6

Chapter 1: Detoxification, the Cornerstone of our Health 7

Chapter 2: The Chemistry of Detoxification 15

Environmental Toxins 16

Self-Generated Toxins.............................18

The Body's Main Organ of Detoxification: The Liver 19

Other Liver Functions That Aid Detoxification......24

Summary 28

Chapter 3: How Diet and Lifestyle Affect Detoxification 29

The Aging Liver..29

Overconsumption of Protein, Fats, and Sugar........32

Prescription, Over-the-Counter, and Recreational Drugs..................................37

Industrial Chemicals...............................39

Medical Conditions................................40

Summary 42

Chapter 4: Detoxification and Peak Performance 43

Physical Vitality and Stamina..........................43

Mental Clarity and Acuity 49

The Ability to Get Along with Other People..........55

The Ability to Remain Calm Under Pressure 68

Summary 73

Chapter 5: Detoxification and Health 75

Cold and Flu-like Symptoms 76
Chronic Fatigue and Environmental Allergies 79
Nervous System Disease 80
Alcohol-Related Heart Disease 81
Elevated Estrogen Levels 82
Sexual Problems 84
Cancer 84

Chapter 6: Evaluating Your Detoxification Ability ...86

Checklist: Do You Have Healthy Detoxification? ..86
Laboratory Tests to Evaluate Liver Function 91
Summary 92

Part II: Restoring Your Ability to Detoxify 94

Chapter 7: Introduction to my Detoxification
Program 95

A Caution on Starting Your Detoxification
Program 96

Chapter 8: The Detoxification Diet 98

More Specific Information on Diet 100

Chapter 9: Modified Fasting 104
Chapter 10: Juice Fasting 108

Cautions on Juice Fasting 109
Guidelines for Juice Fasting 110
Types of Juicers 112
Nutrients Found In Fresh Fruits and Vegetables .115

Chapter 11: Nutritional Supplements to Restore
Detoxification 130

Antioxidants...129
Special Antioxidants 133
Amino Acids 140
Essential Fatty Acids.................................145

Chapter 12: Herbs and Green Foods for Healthy
Detoxification 153

Green Foods 162

Chapter 13: Liver-Cleansing Techniques 169

Using Coffee for a Powerful Detoxification
Technique 170
Liver Flushes..174
Colon Cleanses 176
Therapeutic Baths, Sweats, and Saunas.................180
Summary of Treatment Options for Restoring
Your Ability to Detoxify..............................1877

About Susan Richards, M.D. 188
Notes...189
Notes...191

Part I:
How Detoxification Benefits Peak Performance and Health

1

Detoxification, the Cornerstone of our Health

Detoxification is one of our body's most crucial functions. It refers to the process of neutralizing or transforming substances that would normally be poisonous or harmful, and eliminating them from the body. Without proper detoxification, toxic substances would accumulate within the body and impair our health by interfering with the function of all our vital organ systems.

The liver is our primary organ of detoxification. It is the main interface between both ingested and internally created toxins and all the cells of our bodies. If the liver can handle the toxic load we put on our bodies, we can perform at our best and remain healthy. If liver function is impaired, however, our performance in life, our emotions and health are negatively affected in many different ways.

Poor detoxification function is linked to reacting with inappropriate behavior (usually anger) to many of life's inconsequential annoyances, chronic low-grade fatigue, muddled thinking or brain fog upon arising in the morning. It's linked to many different illnesses, including many female hormone related conditions, allergies, autoimmune diseases, heart disease and even cancer.

I want to share with you the stories of two women that I have seen as patients. Both women had impaired detoxification that affected their health and well-being in very different ways.

Michelle was a woman in her early forties who was suffering from estrogen dominance due, in part, to poor detoxification. She consulted me as a patient because she was facing a possible hysterectomy due to a fibroid tumor that was causing heavy menstrual bleeding. She wanted to avoid surgery as well as treat her uncomfortable PMS symptoms.

When I took Michelle's patient history, I found that one week to ten days out of each month, she was suffering from moderate to severe PMS symptoms. She had an unhealthy high fat, high sugar intake diet, often eating fast foods like pizza, soft drinks, cookies, and ice cream. Her dietary habits were even worse premenstrually when food cravings would increase, along with mood swings, irritability, and bloating.

Her unhealthy diet was definitely affecting her detox-ification ability and was contributing to her estrogen dominance. Research studies have shown that over-indulgence in foods like sugar, alcohol, caffeine and fat can greatly affect the liver's ability to metabolize female hormones.

I recommended that she change her dietary habits significantly since she wanted to avoid a hysterectomy. She was willing to make the necessary changes and began to eat a more nutrient rich, vegetarian emphasis diet. She found that she could still eat foods like tacos, burritos and burgers, but now made with much more healthful ingredients like whole grains and legumes. She also began to eat more salads and steamed vegetables.

In addition, I created for her a powerful program of nutritional supplements to her bring her estrogen dominance under control and support the health of her liver. She began a program of daily exercise, including taking walks and working out at her local gym. The effects were quite dramatic!

Her new detoxification-friendly diet not only eliminated her PMS symptoms but also helped her to lose twenty unwanted pounds as her detoxification ability improved. She was thrilled to find that her heavy menstrual bleeding stopped within a few menstrual cycles and that she no longer needed to have a hysterectomy.

My second story is about my patient, Tanya. She suffered from social anxiety and shared with me that when she went to parties with friends or had get togethers with her co-workers, she drank too much alcohol to reduce her feelings of nervousness. Being a single woman, she was also trying to date since she was interested in having a committed, long-term relationship. She found her first attempts at dating equally difficult and drank too much alcohol to deal with her post-date anxiety.

As her alcohol intake started to affect her detoxification capacity, she began to suffer increasingly more from hangovers and fatigue the morning after drinking too much. The alcohol was also beginning to cause digestive upset and acne breakouts. She was very concerned about her fatigue and hangovers since it was beginning to affect her job performance.

Tanya and I talked at length about feasible solutions for her problem. She felt like she needed a stronger support system, so she decided to join a woman's group at her church and work with a therapist to start managing her social anxiety. She slowly began to cut down on her alcohol intake while starting on a detoxification support program that I created for her. I included in her program nutrients to support and restore the health of her liver as well as reduce her anxiety and create more of a sense of peace and calm. I reinforced these benefits with a diet that helped to balance her brain chemistry and blood sugar level along with providing support for her liver.

She found the program to be very helpful and shared with me that her anxiety was starting to diminish. She was able to attend get-togethers and be comfortable enough socializing to enjoy a non-alcoholic drink. Her energy level picked up as her digestive symptoms and skin breakouts began to resolve. She was clearly on a path back to health and wellness.

Both of these patients demonstrate how important healthy detoxification is to our health and well-being. Unfortunately, Michelle and Tanya are typical of the millions of people in our society who suffer from poor detoxification related illnesses.

Western culture is firmly rooted in the pleasure principle. Many people enjoy eating rich foods, drinking alcoholic beverages, and even smoking to increase their enjoyment of life or as a reward for working hard and accomplishing their goals. The use of cigarettes, drugs, and alcohol is very common in our society in order to reduce the level of stress and buffer us from the fears and anxieties that would otherwise dampen our moods.

Above all else, we value convenience in many areas of our lives, regardless of its cost or possible harmful effects on our health. Western medicine treats most health problems by using drugs to rapidly suppress symptoms that may potentially cause toxic side effects. Other examples of modern conveniences that have potential health hazards include using toxic solvents for cleaning, using pesticides to eliminate insects, or spraying the lawn with herbicides instead of digging out the weeds.

All of the pleasures and conveniences of modern life generate enormous amounts of toxic residues that we ingest or are exposed to on a daily basis through the air we breathe or even take into our bodies through our skin and mucous membranes. In order to remain in good health, the body must break down and eliminate all of these toxins on a continual basis. In addition, the body must similarly process the by-products of its own metabolism, which, if allowed to accumulate in the body, could cause serious illnesses or even death.

I have written this book as a comprehensive guide on detoxification. You will learn how detoxification functions in our bodies, the role of the liver, and the chemistry of detoxification as well as how to evaluate and test your own detoxification capacity.

You will also develop an understanding of the many ways in which detoxification affects our ability to perform in life, our emotions and our health. Most importantly, I share with you my program on how to support and restore healthy detoxification, including diets, nutritional supplements, cleansing techniques, fasting, and much more. I have used these programs with many thousands of patients who, like Michelle and Tanya, have benefitted greatly. I hope that you will find these programs to be of great benefit to you too, in restoring radiant health, energy and wellness.

In the chart that follows, I summarize the benefits of healthy detoxification.

Benefits of Detoxification

Peak-Performance Benefits

- Enhanced mental clarity and acuity
- Increased resistance to illness
- Increased ability to remain calm under pressure
- Increased ability to get along with other people (permits enjoyment of extensive social and business entertaining)
- Increased physical vitality and stamina (helps improve work productivity)

Health Benefits

- Increased resistance to disease
- Reduces cold and flu-like symptoms
- Eliminates toxins from the body
- Restores liver and digestive health
- Reduces the risk of heart disease
- Protects the nervous system and brain from unmetabolized toxins
- Decreases the risk of PMS, fibroid tumors, endometriosis, and breast cancer
- Promotes sexual performance and maintains libido
- Is used as a complementary therapy for the treatment of cancer

Let's get started!

2

The Chemistry of Detoxification

In this chapter, I am going to discuss the different types of toxins that we are constantly exposed to and the incredible process of detoxification that is constantly occurring within our bodies to break down and eliminate these dangerous substances. Detoxification is one of the most important functions within our bodies since it protects us from their negative effects of so many thousands of chemicals.

I will then discuss the process of detoxification itself and how it works within our bodies. Supporting the process of detoxification through safe, all natural healing methods and keeping it working efficiently is one of the most important things that we can do to maintain our health. Let's begin right now!

Two different kinds of toxins must be processed by the body in order to maintain our health: those that are generated in the environment and those that are generated within the body.

Environmental Toxins

Beginning early in this century and accelerating in the last four or five decades, there has been an enormous increase in the number and amount of environmental pollutants that we are exposed to on a daily basis. Our ability to process and excrete these toxins is crucial for survival.

Our bodies are being assaulted on a daily basis by chemicals such as pesticides, herbicides, and contaminants from industrial manufacturing that are in the air, water, and food supply. The amount of toxic chemicals we are exposed to in our environment is staggering.

Each year, the average American is exposed to fourteen pounds of food preservatives, additives, colorings, flavorings, antimicrobial agents, waxes (used to preserve produce), and pesticide and herbicide residues. U.S. production of synthetic pesticides exceeds 1.4 billion pounds a year, and the Environmental Protection Agency (EPA) estimates that there are approximately 70,000 various chemicals in foods, drugs, and pesticides that we may be exposed to, any of which the human body must be prepared to deactivate and remove.

In addition, most of us consume highly processed foods that are laden with artificial chemicals and food additives like MSG (monosodium glutamate), a widely used flavor enhancer; aspartame, an artificial sweetener used in many calorie-reduced foods; and trans fatty acids. Trans fatty acids, which are not found in nature, are polyunsaturated vegetable oils that have been chemically altered by hydrogenation, which converts a fat that is liquid at room temperature into one that is solid, like margarine. All of these artificial chemicals must be detoxified and eliminated by the body.

Toxins also accumulate in the body through the ingestion of addictive substances such as alcohol, caffeine, sugar, and nicotine. Manufacturers promote these addictive substances with billions of dollars of advertising, and many of our social customs support their usage. We have every opportunity to indulge in these substances thanks to daily coffee and cigarette breaks at work and the universal availability of these products in every imaginable channel of distribution.

The body must also detoxify prescription and over-the-counter drugs as well as recreational ones. Drugs are commonly broken down by the liver and eliminated through excretory organs like the kidneys. Many Americans routinely take as many as two to three drugs per day in an attempt to quickly fix a health complaint that is often the result of a poor lifestyle choice. Older Americans have been known to be on ten, twenty, or more different drugs for various ailments. Over time, this puts enormous strain on the liver, our main organ of detoxification. No wonder our livers are overworked and stressed!

Self-Generated Toxins

Beside the toxins we take into our bodies from the outside, our bodies also create endogenous toxins (originating from inside the body), which must also be broken down and eliminated. These are chemicals that we produce internally as by-products of metabolism.

When the detoxification process is working efficiently, these toxins are usually neutralized or excreted without unduly stressing the body. However, if allowed to circulate unaltered through the body, these chemical substances can be highly toxic. For example, when you have a protein-rich meal like a steak dinner, the by-product of the chemical break-down of the protein is ammonia, which is highly toxic if allowed to accumulate in the body.

Normally, ammonia is immediately converted by the liver into a harmless substance called urea that can then be excreted from the body through the kidneys. In patients with severe liver disease, however, this ability to convert ammonia is compromised and ammonia can become elevated to dangerously high levels.

When toxic substances are not properly neutralized and excreted from the body, they are stored in the cells, particularly in fatty tissue. Our cells and tissues can store toxins for months, even years, releasing them during times of low food intake, exercise, or stress. When they are finally released into the bloodstream, the toxins can trigger unwanted symptoms as the body reacts to these poisons, including tiredness, dizziness, nausea, and a racing pulse.

Many chronic and even deadly diseases such as coronary heart disease and diseases of the nervous system, liver, pancreas, and other vital organs have been linked to impaired detoxification. Both the health and performance consequences of poor detox-ification have been corroborated by many research studies.

The Body's Main Organ of Detoxification: The Liver

When the liver is working efficiently, it buffers the body internally from the harmful effects of ingested toxins and environmental pollutants as well as the by-products of our own metabolism. Most people are unaware of the vital role the liver plays in maintaining health, equating it only with a food that tastes good when cooked with onions. However, an understanding of how this vital organ functions is crucial for maintaining high performance levels and overall good health.

The liver is one of the most metabolically active and complex organs in the body. It is the largest organ in your body, normally weighing about four pounds. Its large size reflects the multiple functions it performs. The liver lies in the upper right portion of the abdominal cavity beneath the diaphragm. The liver carries out hundreds, if not thousands, of enzymatic reactions along numerous metabolic pathways, playing a pivotal role in maintaining health.

The liver is so crucial to health that it is the only organ that can completely regenerate itself when part of it is removed or damaged. Up to 25 percent of the liver can be removed and it can still perform its tasks. Moreover, its powers of regeneration are awesome! Within a short period of time, the liver will grow back to its original shape and size.

As harmful chemicals and bacteria circulate through the liver, they pass through a network of blood vessels called the portal system. Unlike other organs of the body, the portal system does not receive blood from the heart. Instead, the liver receives much of its blood directly from the intestinal tract. This allows the liver to process the nutrients and any ingested pollutants before they reach the general circulation. The liver processes about three pints of blood, or an average of 29 percent of a person's total cardiac output, per minute.

The liver deactivates and removes the toxic chemicals that circulate throughout the body by two methods. The first method consists of filtering channels called sinusoids. Cells that line the sinusoids surround and break down foreign debris, bacteria, and toxic chemicals via phagocytosis, the process in which one molecule digests another. The second method consists of an extensive two-step system of enzymes that facilitate the deactivation and elimination of toxins. There are two phases to this process.

Phase I involves a group of enzymes called the cytochrome P-450 system. This system contains between fifty and a hundred enzymes, each of which detoxifies specific types of chemicals. In this phase, toxins undergo oxidation and reduction, in which electrons are transferred between molecules. They are also rendered more water soluble.

Most harmful chemicals, such as pesticides, herbicides, alcohol, and drugs, are fat soluble when they first enter the body, which allows them to be stored in our fatty tissue and therefore makes them more difficult to eliminate from the body. But when toxins are rendered water soluble, they can be more easily excreted through the kidneys and intestinal tract.

Phase I of the detoxification process reduces the toxicity of chemicals that would be harmful to the body if they were allowed to remain in their original state. After this phase, toxins are neutralized, excreted from the body through the intestines or urinary tract, or converted into an intermediate form suitable for further processing by the phase II detoxification system. As these intermediate products are formed, free radicals are generated, and antioxidants are necessary to keep these free radicals from damaging the liver. Because these intermediate products are potentially dangerous, it is important that phase II of detoxification be functioning properly to be able to complete the metabolism of these toxins.

Foods such as broccoli, oranges, Brussels sprouts, dill, tangerines, cabbage, and caraway seeds can support this function. Broccoli, Brussels sprouts, and cabbage contain indole-3-carbinol and oranges, tangerines, dill, and caraway seeds contain limonene, both of which stimulate the phase I detoxification enzymes.

In phase II of the detoxification process, the intermediate compounds generated in phase I are transformed into harmless metabolites (breakdown products) that can then be excreted by the body. Phase II enzymes act directly on some toxic substances through a process called conjugation, in which these substances are bound with a protective compound. This process neutralizes or inactivates the toxins or enables them to be more readily eliminated from the body.

Phase II detoxification occurs through the production of glutathione, a substance composed of three amino acids, cysteine, glutamic acid, and glycine, and other sulfur-containing compounds such as sulfuric and glucurunic acid. Several amino acids, including glycine, glutamine, arginine, ornithine, and taurine, along with acetyl CoA and methyl groups (which originate from the amino acid methionine), also combine with and neutralize toxins in phase II. Conjugation removes toxins from their free state, in which they could ordinarily cause cellular stress or damage. Conjugated toxins are then excreted through the urinary tract or the intestines.

Examples of substances that must be detoxified by the liver are the many hormones produced within the body. Hormones like estrogen, testosterone, adrenaline, and insulin must be efficiently metabolized and excreted from the body. Otherwise, they would accumulate to toxic levels, producing a variety of adverse effects. Hormones circulate throughout the body, being transported in the blood to various tissues and organ systems.

As hormones pass through the liver, they are inactivated by being bound to sulfuric and glucuronic acid and converted to less potent forms. This process of binding hormones with other chemicals makes them unable to attach to the specific hormone receptor sites within the cells. Once hormones have been detoxified by the liver, they are then secreted with the bile into the small intestine and eliminated through the bowels.

The detoxification of alcohol also occurs in the liver. Detoxification lessens the toxic effects of alcohol on the liver by helping to convert the alcohol into less harmful end products. When this process does not function properly, alcohol residues can cause serious inflammatory changes within the liver. Many medications, insecticides, heavy metals, and nicotine from cigarette smoke are examples of other toxic substances treated by phase II detoxification.

Other Liver Functions That Aid Detoxification

The liver performs many other important functions that assist in and support the process of detoxification. These include the liver's production of bile as well as its functions as a storage reservoir for blood and as a filter of bacteria and viruses. The liver also aids in the digestion, absorption, storage, and utilization of many vitamins, minerals, protein, sugar, and fat. While not specifically needed for detoxification, these other functions are all crucial for the maintenance of peak performance and good health.

Bile production

The liver produces bile, a yellowish-green fluid that is stored in the gallbladder and secreted into the intestine to emulsify (disperse into smaller droplets) and facilitate the digestion of fats. Toxins are also secreted into the bile and then eliminated from the body through the intestinal tract. Thus, adequate bile production helps to reduce the workload of the liver.

Within the liver, bile is transported through small ducts into larger canals and, finally, into the gallbladder where it is stored and concentrated. Lecithin, the emulsifying agent in the bile, transforms large fat globules into tiny ones, which are more water soluble and more readily assimilated. Bile helps the body excrete breakdown products from the blood, neutralizes stomach acid, promotes intestinal peristalsis, and increases the absorption of the fat-soluble vitamins, A, D, E, and K.

Blood storage

Since the liver is an organ that can expand and contract, it is capable of serving as a reservoir for blood when there is excess volume in circulation. It is also capable of supplying extra blood to the rest of the body when blood volume is low. The normal blood volume of the liver is about 10 percent of the body's total blood volume.

Only one-quarter of the blood that circulates through the liver is derived from general circulation; the remaining three-quarters comes from the portal blood flow, which is derived from the intestines, stomach, spleen, and pancreas. This portal blood carries bacteria picked up from the intestines. The liver is said to cleanse this blood through the action of cells within the liver that digest and destroy these bacteria.

The proper release of blood from the liver is critical for good health. The liver is also involved in the formation of blood, creating serum proteins such as albumin, which maintain fluid balance through osmosis and act as transport molecules. Traditional Asian medicine has long recognized the importance of the liver's blood storage function, using terms such as "blood deficiency" and "blood stagnancy" to explain the origins of various health problems. For example, visual problems, muscle spasms, and menstrual-bleeding abnormalities are all diagnosed in terms of liver blood flow.

Virus and bacteria filtration

Blood flowing through the intestinal capillaries picks up many bacteria from the intestines. Within the liver, the Kupffer cells line the hepatic sinuses. These cells engulf and digest about 99 percent of the bacteria present. Only the remaining 1 percent of the bacteria escapes destruction within the liver and is able to pass through the liver into the general circulation.

Bacteria and yeast can also form toxins that are absorbed into the bloodstream and carried throughout the body. These microbes are implicated in various diseases, including ulcerative colitis, thyroid disease, allergies, and immune disorders. The healthy liver filters out these pathogens, further reducing stress on the immune system.

Other Important Functions of the Liver

Besides its detoxification functions, the liver also plays an important role in the metabolism of protein, fat, and carbohydrates. In addition, numerous compounds essential to the growth, repair, and maintenance of body tissues are either stored or manufactured in the liver, including glucose, cholesterol, and lipoproteins. Many important nutrients are also stored in the liver, including the vitamins A, D, E, and B12; and the minerals iron and copper. Healthy liver function is also necessary to regulate the blood sugar level.

Summary

The liver plays a pivotal role in maintaining health. It performs so many functions and is so crucial to the body that it is the only organ that can completely regenerate itself. The liver is the main organ of detoxification, cleansing the blood of harmful chemicals, viruses, and bacteria; it produces bile, which is essential in the digestion of fat; it stores extra blood; it helps to metabolize protein, fat, and carbohydrates; and it stores important nutrients.

3

How Diet and Lifestyle Affect Detoxification

Given the liver's crucial role as our primary organ of detoxification, any physical or chemical stress that decreases its ability to carry out this function will strongly compromise many aspects of performance and health.

Fortunately, many of these stressors are due to lifestyle habits that we control. By supporting liver function through healthy lifestyle practices, one can maintain the ability to detoxify at effective and peak levels well into old age.

The Aging Liver

The decrease in the liver's detoxification capability is not readily apparent in standard medical testing. While the liver does go through some structural changes as the body ages, these changes consist of only minor alterations, a slight shrinking in the size of the liver and some changes in cell structure. This decrease in size parallels a similar decrease in overall body size, a process that continues from age fifty to seventy.

However, research studies show no significant alterations with age in the most common laboratory indicators of liver function, serum bilirubin, serum glutamic pyruvic transaminase (SGPT), serum glutamic oxaloacetic transaminase (SGOT), and which are all low in people with normal liver function. Hepatic blood flow does decline somewhat with age, but only with the normal decrease in cardiac output.

However, declines in the liver's detoxification capability do occur in some individuals and are often accelerated by external factors related to exposure to environmental toxins and lifestyle habits. These include lack of B vitamins, infectious disease, overconsumption of alcohol, overuse of drugs, and exposure to industrial chemicals. Over time, the cumulative effect of these toxins can cause chronic liver damage.

Alcohol

The most common cause of liver stress and damage in the United States today is the overconsumption of alcohol. It is estimated that more than 100 million Americans consume alcoholic beverages. When the liver's ability to detoxify alcohol is overwhelmed, peak-performance capability is significantly diminished. Moreover, chronic overconsumption can cause inflammatory changes within the liver, which can finally lead to fibrosis and permanent damage to the liver's cells. As many as a million liver cells can be destroyed by a single alcoholic drink.

Numerous research studies document the specific ways in which alcohol impairs liver function. Habitual overconsumption of alcohol can increase the risk of developing a number of degenerative diseases, including hepatitis and cirrhosis, as well as nerve and brain dysfunction, gastritis and ulcers, pancreatitis, hypoglycemia, diabetes, gout, immune suppression, and some types of cancer. The overconsumption of alcohol also increases a person's susceptibility to other toxins such as carbon tetrachloride. It has been estimated that the overconsumption of alcohol can shorten a person's life span by ten to fifteen years.

People who regularly drink alcoholic beverages are particularly susceptible to multiple vitamin and mineral deficiencies. Because alcohol contains very few nutrients and also suppresses appetite, a person drinking alcohol eats less and takes in fewer vitamins and minerals. Finally, the alcohol molecule is small and easy to absorb, so it is preferentially assimilated before other, more nutrient-rich foods can be metabolized.

Alcohol consumption also leads to an increase in daily caloric intake. One ounce of hard liquor is 80 calories, five ounces of wine 100 calories, twelve ounces of beer 140 calories, and various mixed drinks made with juices, sodas, and sweeteners can be between 100 and 250 calories. The average social drinker obtains 5 to 10 percent of their calories from alcohol, while alcoholics may consume more than 50 percent of their calories as alcohol. The empty (meaning, nutrient-poor) calories in alcohol can also lead to weight gain, especially as the toxins in alcohol disrupt fat metabolism.

While alcohol adds significant calories to the diet, it simultaneously impairs digestion and absorption of many nutrients from the small intestine, including the fat-soluble vitamins, A, D, E, and K, plus thiamine, vitamin B6, vitamin B12, choline, folic acid, and some minerals.

Alcohol has a diuretic effect as well, promoting the excretion of nutrients in the urine. Numerous studies document the close correlation between alcohol intake and specific nutrient deficiencies. Alcoholics frequently show low levels of beta-carotene, zinc, thiamine, and vitamin B6. Magnesium deficiency often occurs in chronic alcoholics due to increased loss of magnesium through the urinary tract, which is exacerbated by magnesium deficiency in the diet.

Overconsumption of Protein, Fats, and Sugar

The standard American diet abounds with foods high in protein, fats, and sugar, everything from milk shakes and hamburgers to filet mignon and cherry cheesecake. These foods place tremendous stress on the liver, which has to process them and convert their residue into waste products that can be eliminated from the body.

One indication that the liver is not handling this task adequately is poor digestion. Common signs are gas pains, a feeling of fullness or bloating in the stomach and intestines, marked distaste for oily foods, loss of appetite, constipation (less than one bowel movement per day), and soreness in the liver under moderate fingertip pressure. Many of my patients suffer from poor detoxification and, as a result, often complain about common symptoms of indigestion.

Protein

Only a finite amount of protein can accumulate within the cells of the body. Once the cells have been filled to their limit, excess amino acids are degraded by the liver so that they can be either used as a source of energy or stored as fat. This degradation begins with a process called deamination.

Ammonia, a toxic by-product similar to the ammonia in bottled cleaning solutions, is generated during this process. Ammonia is a strong-smelling and extremely potent poison. In order to avoid the accumulation of toxic levels of ammonia in the blood, the liver metabolizes it into urea, a harmless substance that can be eliminated via the kidneys.

When a person's diet is very high in protein, though, more ammonia is generated and the liver must work harder to metabolize it. Ammonia will accumulate in the blood of individuals with severe liver disease; this accumulation is toxic to the brain and can lead to coma.

Fats

The high fat content of the American diet contributes approximately 40 percent of all calories consumed. This excessive amount of fat in the diet stresses the liver by adding to its workload. The liver must process the fat, converting it into fuel and various building blocks of the cells such as cholesterol and phospholipids. The liver must also produce bile to help break down the excess fat to prepare it for excretion.

Some of the saturated fats that we consume are converted into hormones such as estrogen, which the liver must eventually deactivate. Specifically, diets high in the saturated fats found in red meat and dairy products tend to promote high levels of estrogen in the body and increase the detoxification load on the liver.

Research studies have shown that vegetarian women eating a low-fat, high-fiber diet excrete two to three times more estrogen in their bowel movements and have 50 percent lower blood levels of estrogen than women eating a diet high in dairy and animal fats.

In addition, large amounts of dietary fat can stress the liver indirectly by causing excessive amounts of estrogen to be reabsorbed from the intestinal tract into the general circulation, thereby increasing the amount of estrogen that the liver must detoxify.

Research studies done at Tufts University Medical School found that the composition of the diet strongly affected the type of bacteria present in the intestinal tract. A high-fat diet promoted the growth of intestinal bacteria that secrete an enzyme called beta-glucuronidase. The estrogen that has been bound and deactivated by the liver can be cleaved by this enzyme.

As a result, it is reconverted back into free estrogen. Estrogen can then be reabsorbed back into the general circulation, thereby increasing the estrogen load that the liver must metabolize. In contrast, a diet low in fat and high in fiber promotes the excretion of estrogen from the body, decreasing the amount circulating through the body — and, in particular, the liver.

Sugar

Sugar stored in the liver can also impair its function. Yet Americans eat an extraordinary amount of refined sugar and the quantity continues to rise. According to the Economic Research Service of the USDA, U.S. consumption of total caloric sweeteners was 128.6 pounds per capita in 1986, and continued to rise to 154.5 pounds per capita several decades later.

When the liver stores too much glucose as well as toxins, the canals through which bile flows can become compressed, which decreases bile flow and impairs digestion. Excess stored glucose therefore makes the liver work harder to produce bile and essential digestive enzymes.

A research study published in *The American Journal of Medicine* documented signs of possible liver injury associated with the typical high-sugar American diet. Twenty-one normal adult males consumed a typical diet containing 25 to 30 percent sucrose for eighteen days and a "calorically diluted" diet containing less than 10 percent sucrose for twelve days. Levels of SGOT and SGPT, two enzymes that are released from liver cells into the bloodstream when these cells are acutely damaged, rose significantly when the men were on the high-sucrose diet and returned to baseline levels when they were on the low-sucrose diet.

Prescription, Over-the-Counter, and Recreational Drugs

Frequent use of medications causes the liver to work overtime in order to metabolize them. When drugs are used in moderation and the liver is healthy, it can normally detoxify them quite efficiently. However, when large amounts of medication or recreational drugs are ingested, especially when combined with other toxic substances such as alcohol, these substances can easily overwhelm the liver's detoxification ability.

Although over-the-counter (OTC) products such as anti-inflammatory medications are usually less toxic than prescription drugs, they are also more frequently abused, since they can be readily obtained without visiting a doctor and are less expensive. In America, there are over 50 million regular users of aspirin, with 20 to 25 billion tablets taken each year. Though most consumers usually consider OTC drugs harmless, the excessive use of them can cause dangerous side effects and even be life threatening — in part because the liver's ability to detoxify them is overwhelmed.

An interesting case study, published in *The Journal of Family Practice*, noted the history of a thirty-seven-year-old closet drinker who was taking multiple OTC and prescription medications. After taking a cough medication for an upper-respiratory infection, she arrived in the emergency room with significantly elevated liver enzymes. The patient was given intensive support but died ten hours later. In this tragic case, the chemically overloaded liver was unable to clear the cough medication rapidly enough from her body. As a result, her body went into a state of toxic overload.

Recreational drugs, including cocaine, speed, crack, opium, methadone, and heroin, are particularly toxic to the liver. Substances such as THC (the active ingredient in marijuana) and nicotine remain in the body for several weeks or even months.

Certain prescription drugs have well-documented side effects involving the liver. For example, the use of cimetidine (Tagamet), an antiulcer medication, may result in liver damage in susceptible individuals. Older people are particularly susceptible to the toxic effects that medications may have on liver function: Not only have they cumulatively taken more medications in their lifetime, in general, but they also typically consume more prescription and over-the-counter medications than younger people.

One of my patients, Rose, had severe liver impairment and suffered from excruciating pain due to inflammation of the liver. Her physician placed her on morphine to handle the pain. Rose worked with me to clean up her very unhealthy diet and began a powerful, all natural liver support program of nutritional supplements. She was gradually able to cut back on her morphine dosage, which in itself was toxic to her liver, and finally discontinued it altogether. I am pleased to report that Rose is now drug free and her level of pain is much diminished. Her overall health and the health of her liver is greatly improved and she has much more energy and stamina than she previously had.

Industrial Chemicals

In the normal course of the day, we may be exposed to extremely toxic chemicals on the job and in the products we buy. For instance, chlorinated solvents such as carbon tetrachloride and chlorobenzene are used for degreasing and cleaning many types of machinery. Furniture strippers that contain chlorinated solvents may have been used on woodwork in your home.

Chlorinated solvents can also strip the naturally protective oils from the skin, lung tissue, and eyes, causing damage on the cellular level. These solvents in drinking water have also been associated with chronic liver problems, as well as weakness of the kidney and heart. They are also suspected of causing certain types of cancer. Such chronic exposure to this myriad of chemical substances will, over time, weaken the liver's detoxification capability.

Medical Conditions

Some medical conditions affect the liver's ability to detoxify, including a vitamin B deficiency and hepatitis. Cirrhosis of the liver is the most serious, and usually fatal, liver disease.

Vitamin B deficiency

Vitamin B complex plays a special role in maintaining liver health. When there is a deficiency of the B vitamins, a person's ability to detoxify is greatly hindered. A deficiency of vitamin B complex and its link to liver disease was first researched in the 1940's by Morton S. Biskind, in both animal and human studies.

In an animal research study published in 1942 in *Endocrinology*, Dr. Biskind demonstrated that a B-complex deficiency could impair the liver's ability to deactivate a form of estrogen. Furthermore, Biskind noted that female patients with signs and symptoms of vitamin B deficiency also suffered from symptoms of excessive estrogen such as menorrhagia (heavy menstrual bleeding), premenstrual tension, and chronic cystic mastitis (painful breasts). He found that supplementation with B vitamins such as thiamine, riboflavin, and niacin helped to resolve the symptoms of excessive estrogen.

Hepatitis and cirrhosis

Hepatitis is an inflammatory disease of the liver that can be caused by exposure to a virus, chemical toxins such as alcohol or drugs, tainted food, or a blockage of the duct leading from the liver to the gallbladder. Symptoms of hepatitis include nausea, vomiting, jaundice, loss of appetite, tenderness in the upper-right abdomen, aching muscles, and joint pain.

While many individuals do recover from hepatitis and, over time, even regain normal liver function, not everyone does. In certain individuals, hepatitis does not resolve, and chronic liver disease develops. This often occurs with long-term exposure to pathogens like viruses. With end-stage liver disease, a condition called cirrhosis develops in which the inflammation of liver cells gradually leads to damage of cell structure. The gradual loss of liver function results, as living cells become surrounded by pockets of scar tissue, thereby shutting off the flow of portal blood to the remaining healthy tissue.

As mentioned earlier, liver cells have the capacity to regenerate following many forms of illness, but cirrhosis is not one of them. Cirrhosis is usually fatal, as toxins accumulate in the body. It can be caused by anything from ingestion of toxic chemicals such as carbon tetrachloride, to viral diseases such as infectious hepatitis, to infectious processes in the bile ducts. However, alcoholism is the most common cause.

Summary

A variety of dietary and lifestyle factors can harm the liver, including the overconsumption of alcohol, protein, fats, sugar, and drugs. Toxic chemicals in the environment are also harmful. Changes in lifestyle can eliminate or greatly limit these stressors, as the liver responds well to a healthy lifestyle, and aging does not greatly affect its detoxification capacity.

4

Detoxification and Peak Performance

A properly functioning liver can greatly assist you in performing at a peak level and attaining many of your goals and aspirations. This is because healthy detoxification helps us to maintain a high level of physical energy, our cognitive function, the ability to make sound decisions, and the ability to remain calm during times of stress.

It also helps us to maintain healthy business and social relationships by allowing us to enjoy social situations without any limitation on the types of food and drink we can ingest. Individuals who need to restrict their food intake can undoubtedly survive at social occasions, dinner, and banquets where choice is minimal, but their options may be few.

Physical Vitality and Stamina

Success in most areas of life requires a tremendous amount of physical energy and stamina—this cannot be maintained without a healthy detoxification capability. Most people are unaware of the crucial role that detoxification plays in maintaining one's level of energy.

However, all of us have witnessed individuals who maintain their level of energy, even under adverse circumstances, because their detoxification capability is functioning effectively. These are the people who can work all day with pollutant-laden recirculated air in hermetically sealed office buildings and still feel energetic and fresh at the end of the workday. Unlike many millions of chemically-sensitive people, these individuals seem to be impervious to the chemical pollutants commonly found in such environments, such as benzene, formaldehyde, and toluene.

Several of our modern sealed buildings with their synthetic carpeting and furnishings expose their occupants to high levels of such toxic chemicals. Only with a well-functioning detoxification capability can they thrive and maintain their physical energy and stamina after years of exposure to such toxic environments.

In addition, these same individuals are often able to eat rich food accompanied by fine wines, drink at social and business affairs, and generally expose themselves to a wide variety of pollutants that the body must detoxify. Yet, because they have inherently strong liver function, they are able to detoxify all of these pollutants and continue to have a tremendously high level of energy.

The millions of Americans who do not have well-functioning detoxification systems, however, take daily hits to their energy and stamina because they are unable to efficiently metabolize the vast ocean of toxic chemicals in which we are all immersed.

Morning grogginess and brain fog are a daily concern for many of us, because toxins accumulate during the night and are not broken down by the liver and eliminated from the body. When the liver is unable to detoxify efficiently, the toxic substances generated within the body while a person is asleep are not fully metabolized until later in the day, after the liver has become more active. This can lead to a slow start in the morning.

The tendency to feel tired and groggy is even greater if a person has eaten a heavy meal or consumed alcoholic beverages late the night before. Many people need that first cup of morning coffee to clear their head and restore their physical energy. They will drink coffee throughout the morning, until their liver has finally cleared the accumulated toxic load. Some of my patients report that they drink as many as four to six cups of coffee or other caffeinated beverages in the morning; this consumption then tapers off in the afternoon, once their energy level picks up.

I have found that poor liver detoxification is often an important causal factor in patients who complain of chronic fatigue. Some of these patients also have symptoms of poor liver function or even a history of prior liver disease such as hepatitis. Symptoms of digestive distress due to poor liver function—such as bloating, discomfort in the upper-right abdominal area, and the inability to tolerate rich or fatty foods—can be seen in these patients. They also tend to be intolerant of alcohol. If they are women, they may also suffer from many common female problems such as PMS, heavy and/or irregular menstrual flow, and fibroid tumors of the uterus due, in part, to their liver's inability to detoxify estrogen.

Many of those with poor detoxification capability complain about underperforming in important areas of their lives because they simply lack the physical energy and vitality to do so. These people are genuinely upset by their inability to participate in many of the joys of living. I have found that many of these individuals benefit greatly from a liver detoxification program of the type described in the next chapter. Once the liver's detoxification ability is restored, they are able to reduce their dependence on stimulants while regaining their physical energy and stamina.

A good example is Christine, a local real-estate agent who was in her late forties when she first consulted me about her chronic fatigue. During her twenty-year career, Christine always had sufficient energy to perform the many functions required of realtors.

Success in the real-estate business requires a great amount of physical energy: Realtors are expected to be available to show houses at any time of the day or night, including weekends. There are constant tours, open houses, staff and client meetings. Negotiations between the buyer and seller are often highly stressful, with deals sometimes falling through after weeks of effort.

As part of her work, Christine enjoyed socializing frequently with her clients and coworkers. She would often enjoy a glass or two of wine after work and continued to drink into the evening at the social events she attended three to four nights a week.

However, in the year before her consultation with me, Christine began to find the physical demands of her job difficult to meet. To sustain her flagging energy, she began to increase her coffee intake significantly, starting with a mug of black coffee as soon as she got out of bed. She even kept a thermos in her car so she could get a caffeine boost while driving.

Upon evaluation, I found that Christine's liver function tests were mildly elevated, probably due to her overconsumption of alcohol. She also had many symptoms typical of compromised liver function, such as bloating after eating fatty food and mild abdominal discomfort. Given all of these facts, I recommended that Christine begin a liver-cleansing program as well as reduce her intake of alcohol and fatty foods.

Over a period of several months, Christine noted an improvement in her level of energy and was able to decrease her dependence on caffeine down to one cup of coffee per day, which she used for enjoyment rather than as a necessity.

Blood tests to assess the health of the liver are often normal or only mildly elevated until the liver is severely damaged from alcohol abuse, illness, or toxic chemical exposure. The ability of the liver to detoxify may be greatly reduced, yet standard medical tests may still be within the normal range.

If you suspect that you have compromised liver function based on symptoms of fatigue, inability to process moderate amounts of alcohol, abdominal bloating, intolerance to fatty foods, and needing to drink significant amounts of coffee to get started in the morning, it may be helpful to try the liver-strengthening suggestions described later on in this book. Try them for a month or two to see if your symptoms begin to diminish. If so, you may want to maintain a liver restoration program until your symptoms improve further. If you do not notice any benefit, however, your problem may not be liver related. In any case, consult with your own physician for a proper diagnostic evaluation.

Mental Clarity and Acuity

The excessive ingestion of alcohol has deleterious effects on cognitive thinking. Millions of Americans are either alcohol abusers or consume alcohol beyond their ability to metabolize it effectively. This can cause significant impairment of their mental sharpness and ability to think clearly. Most people have experienced, at least to some degree, the negative effect that alcohol has on cognitive function. Anyone who has had a drink and become mildly inebriated has experienced the mild signs of toxicity — blurred thinking and a slight lack of coordination. Because alcohol is rapidly absorbed and can cross the blood-brain barrier, the effect is felt rapidly.

Most teenagers and young adults can more easily metabolize all the alcohol they consume. I remember men friends in college, with prodigious detoxification capability, who could drink large quantities of beer at night and still show up for early classes clearheaded and do well on exams.

However, most people, by the time they reach their thirties and forties, can no longer drink with abandon and still perform high-level cognitive functions. Beyond the fifth decade, it is only individuals with super functioning detoxification systems who can continue to consume large amounts of alcohol and still function as peak performers intellectually.

Numerous research studies have shown that elevated levels of alcohol have a direct toxic effect on the brain and nervous system. For example, research studies have found significant degenerative changes in the brains of chronic alcohol abusers compared to non-alcoholics. One such study, published in *The Lancet*, compared the brains of fifty-five chronic alcoholics with those of eleven non-alcoholics at autopsy. The study confirmed that the brains of alcoholics suffer much more degenerative damage, losing white matter, the part of the brain consisting mainly of nerve fibers.

Frequent alcohol consumption that continues into midlife and beyond may begin to cause an impairment of cognitive abilities, because alcohol becomes more difficult to metabolize with age. Many studies confirm that chronic alcoholics, who have lost their detoxification abilities over the years, score poorly in cognitive testing. One such study, published in *ACTA Neurologica Scandinavica*, stated that 50 to 70 percent of chronic alcoholics exhibit mild to moderate cognitive impairment. This study compared cognitive deterioration in 54 chronic alcoholics as compared to 30 non-alcoholics. Researchers found that alcoholics had significantly lower intellectual and visual-spatial scores than the non-alcoholics.

When a person drinks beyond their ability to process alcohol over a long period of time, the intellectual skills required for their work can be impaired and careers eventually ruined. A good example of this is Frank, a business acquaintance of my family, who used to be a much sought after consulting engineer. He was known for his ability to accurately assess a construction project, prioritize activities, and finish the job on time. But his drinking destroyed his formerly crisp, linear thinking.

As he continued to drink and his health deteriorated, Frank began to make basic technical mistakes in his work. Equipment installations that should have been easy began to go awry. Frank submitted incoherent, disorganized written reports, used exceptionally poor judgment in business situations, and finished projects late. However, he failed to make the connection between his excessive drinking and his diminished mental capabilities. Frank continued his excessive overconsumption of alcohol; and over time, he lost his consulting business and his life's savings. His health also continued to deteriorate.

The brain and nervous system are sensitive to the negative effects of other toxins besides alcohol. Petrochemical-based pollutants such as pesticides, herbicides, and the thousands of industrial and household chemicals to which we are all exposed can also affect cognitive function. These chemicals are fat soluble and tend to accumulate in the brain and nervous system, which are predominantly made up of fats or lipids. Exposure to these pollutants can slow our thought processes and hamper both logical thinking and creative abilities. In addition, many chemicals form metabolites that will also impair one's ability to concentrate, causing symptoms like brain fog and dizziness, if not properly detoxified.

One example is a toxic chemical called trichloroethylene, used as an industrial solvent, which forms a metabolite in the body called chlorhydrate. It can cause significant brain fog and fatigue in susceptible individuals. Common chemicals found in new homes or office furnishings and building materials, such as styrene, toluene, xylene, and formalehyde, can release a significant amount of gas into the indoor environment, causing an inability to concentrate, spaciness, and fatigue.

In addition, individuals working in beauty salons, research laboratories, and dry-cleaning establishments are exposed to these types of toxic chemicals daily. I remember having had significant exposure to chemicals such as toluene and formaldehyde both as a teenager and as a college student working in a medical laboratory, as well as during my years of medical training. At that time, I had no idea how destructive to the liver these chemicals were and did not take precautions. I went through a bout of fatigue during my early practice years and suspected that the accumulated residues of these chemicals may have contributed to my tiredness. I placed myself on a liver detoxification program and, happily, found that both my physical and mental energy were greatly restored!

I've had many patients who have complained about impairment of their cognitive function, both from exposure to chemical pollutants in the workplace and from exposure to toxins released by building materials and furnishings in the home.

My patient, Elizabeth, moved into an apartment that had recently been refurbished with new carpeting, curtains, and furniture, all of which were made from synthetic materials. After moving in, she immediately began to suffer from brain fog, fatigue, and dizziness as well as a constant runny nose. Recognizing that the chemicals emanating from the new furnishings were probably causing her symptoms, she began to stay with friends and found new housing as quickly as possible. Her symptoms resolved as soon as she was no longer living in a toxic environment.

Another patient, Stephanie, reported feeling weak, nauseated, and unable to think clearly whenever she walked near lawns that had recently been sprayed with herbicides. And yet another patient, Maria, had to quit her job as an administrative assistant because she could not handle the toxic load of chemicals that she was exposed to in the hermetically sealed office building in which she worked.

All of these individuals noted impaired cognitive function from exposure to environmental chemicals that their livers were unable to effectively detoxify. They all had to either change location or avoid contact with these offending chemicals. In addition, they began to follow nutritional and cleansing programs to restore their liver's detoxification ability and build up their resistance to those environmental chemicals that we are all inevitably exposed to.

If at all possible, avoid living or working in an environment where you are constantly breathing air-borne pollutants. If you are buying or renting a new home or apartment and suffer from chemical sensitivities, find out if new carpets or furnishings have recently been installed. Often, these are made of synthetic materials that can release toxic gases into the indoor environment.

One of the most effective ways to eliminate airborne petrochemical-based pollutants, viruses, bacteria, mold, fungi, or just plain unpleasant odors is through the use of an ozone generator (ozone is an activated form of oxygen). Portable ozone generators are available for home or office, and corporations should investigate the use of large-scale ones to protect office workers in sealed buildings or in factories where they are working with toxic chemicals. They are available for purchase through the Internet.

The Ability to Get Along with Other People

The social consequences of poor detoxification touch our lives in many ways. The newspapers are full of stories about accidents caused by road rage, violent crimes, and acrimonious litigation. There appears to be an increase in aggressive behavior in our society. Inconsequential and minor behavioral actions, such as the minor driving errors that sometimes trigger road rage, are being met with increasingly hostile reactions.

An article published in *The San Francisco Chronicle* provided statistics assembled by the National Highway Traffic Safety Administration on road rage and the frequency of motor-vehicle fatalities. According to this federal agency, aggressive behaviors were factors in nearly 28,000 of the 42,000 highway deaths each year, and the problem is getting worse. Antisocial behaviors included tailgating, weaving through busy lanes, honking or screaming at other drivers, exchanging insults, using angry hand signs, speeding, changing lanes illegally, running red lights, and even gunfire.

While several factors are involved in every car crash, rage is involved in two-thirds of the deaths and one-third of the nonfatal crashes, resulting in 3 million injuries. In addition, according to *The San Francisco Chronicle* article, the AAA Foundation for Traffic Safety's study of 10,000 aggressive-driving accidents estimated that in 35 percent of cases, a vehicle was used directly as a weapon.

The explosive emotions and violence associated with poor liver function are even expressed through art, books, movies, and TV shows. One of the most noted writers of the 1950s and 1960s, Allen Ginsberg, had a lifetime history of liver disease. Ginsberg made a successful career writing poems full of anger and defiance, including a book of free verse, *Howl and Other Poems*, which is considered the preeminent poetic work of the Beat movement of the 1950s. Ginsberg suffered for many years from hepatitis C, which eventually led to cirrhosis of the liver. He was later diagnosed with cancer of the liver, and he died in 1997 from cardiopulmonary arrest with secondary liver disease.

Poor detoxification capability, at the interpersonal interaction level, affects relationships at the business and personal level. While some employees clearly have emotional or character disorders that make them difficult to work with, the inability to detoxify efficiently can also wreak havoc on one's ability to maintain productive relationships in the workplace and personal life. For example, a liver that is grossly malfunctioning due to substance abuse such as alcohol or drug addiction can cause an individual to behave in an abusive or aggressive manner toward their co-workers.

This issue is typified by the predicament of a patient I saw some years ago. Cassie is a young scientist who had recently begun to work in a large research facility. She initially consulted me because of chest pain and headaches, which turned out to be stress related. Cassie's work situation was particularly difficult, in that her supervisor disliked her and made her work life miserable with constant criticism. She also gave Cassie so much extra paperwork that she had to spend outside time to complete it. The fact that Cassie heard from other employees that this supervisor was "difficult" for everyone to deal with was of no consolation to her.

Luckily for Cassie, the vice president, who had been protecting and even encouraging her supervisor's behavior left the company. The new vice president was informed by other employees about the supervisor's inappropriate and demoralizing behavior.

Upon looking into the situation, he found that her behavior toward Cassie and others was unacceptable; and he also discovered that she was a closet alcoholic. Having determined that she was a real liability for the company, harming both morale and productivity, he terminated her from the job.

Traditionally, organizations have dealt with difficult and disruptive personality traits in their employees or members by firing them or requiring them to undergo psychological counseling. There has rarely been any recognition that an individual's aberrant behavior may have biochemical origins.

The importance of making this distinction between a biochemical and a psychiatric disorder is particularly crucial for employees who have performed well previously. If an individual's behavior, which had previously been acceptable, suddenly begins to deviate from their past performance, and there are no obvious stress factors to explain it (such as divorce, illness, death in the family, or financial reversal), the individual should be advised that their problem could be biochemically based and should promptly be evaluated by a physician.

I often see the negative effects of poor detoxification on relationships within my patients' families. Alcohol abuse can be a major cause of upset between family members, resulting in toxic relationships that often end in break-ups or divorce. Further, the children of alcoholics may suffer abuse, both mental and physical, from their alcoholic parents and may need to spend years in support groups trying to recover from the damage.

One example of how impaired liver detoxification can adversely affect family relationships is in women who suffer from premenstrual syndrome (PMS). The single most common problem that these women complain of is the emotional changes they experience premenstrually — and the deterioration of social relationships that these changes can cause.

Research studies have suggested that there is a close relationship between PMS and the liver's ability to detoxify hormones efficiently. This link was first noted sixty years ago by Morton S. Biskind, who discovered the liver is responsible for detoxifying estrogen.

Elevated estrogen levels during the second half of the menstrual cycle are thought to predispose women to PMS symptoms, since it is known that estrogen affects brain function and is a strong determinant of mood. Elevated estrogen levels have been linked to such common PMS symptoms as anxiety, panic attacks, irritability, and mood swings.

Biskind's initial studies, on both laboratory animals and human beings, found that the liver is responsible for detoxifying and inactivating estrogen as it circulates through the body in the bloodstream. Poor liver function can lead to elevated levels of estrogen, thereby increasing the tendency toward PMS.

My PMS patients often describe themselves as short-tempered, grouchy, and highly critical. Studies that discuss the behavioral changes that occur in women with PMS have found that the aberrant behavior varies from milder symptoms of poor social function to antisocial and highly destructive behavior. In women with severe PMS, marital conflict is common. Some women even complain about their tendency to abuse their children, emotionally and physically, during their premenstrual period.

Women may develop phobias and sleep disturbances for one or two weeks out of the month, and they may experience depression and lethargy. At the far end of the spectrum, various studies demonstrate that women tend to have high rates of aberrant behavior, psychiatric episodes, and even crimes of passion during their premenstrual phase.

Because alcohol is a known liver toxin, women with PMS may be particularly susceptible to its deleterious effects. This link was evaluated in a study published in *Obstetrics and Gynecology*. Researchers evaluated two separate groups of women, 95 who received treatment for PMS and 147 who did not. The women were screened for alcoholism and were assessed using a questionnaire followed by an interview.

The researchers found that 72 percent of the PMS patients had a history of alcohol abuse, as compared with only 45 percent of the non-PMS sufferers. Women with PMS may be equally intolerant of other foods that compromise liver function, such as saturated fats and refined sugar.

One of the first steps that I often take in treating my PMS patients is to recommend a liver-cleansing program. This helps to restore the liver's detoxification capability and allows the liver to metabolize hormones, such as estrogen, more efficiently.

The benefits of a liver restoration program begin to be evident within a few weeks. Often, within several menstrual cycles, PMS sufferers report that their moods are substantially improved. Women with families state that they have more patience in dealing with their children and are able to stop themselves before they begin to bicker with their husbands or significant others during the premenstrual period. They also report more socially appropriate behavior and are more even tempered at work or with friends.

Healthy liver function and social entertaining

Another benefit of having healthy detoxification function is being able to fully participate in many different types of social events, such as receptions and dinner parties, where food and drink are part of the hospitality. Invariably, alcohol is served as well as foods high in fat, such as canapés, cheeses, heavy sauces on entrées, and rich desserts. A person with optimal detoxification capability can enjoy this food and drink with no ill effects. However, someone with marginal liver detoxification capability may instinctively avoid much of what is being served, or will indulge and then pay the penalty the next day, with fatigue, brain fog, or even inappropriate behavior.

For many politicians, corporate executives, public relations personnel, brokers, agents, and sales reps, the ability to entertain clients often and to eat and drink without fear of a severe hangover or energy drop can be a prerequisite for career success. In addition, many people like to go out informally for dinner or after work with coworkers whose company they enjoy.

The individual who can share a convivial drink with coworkers, clients, and customers is perceived as mixing well with others and being more socially accessible. Again, I am referring to someone who can manage their alcohol intake, uses it as a social facilitator, and, of course, knows when to quit, not someone who becomes habitually over intoxicated

Of course, there are also many people who work nine-to-five jobs, whether schoolteachers, hospital personnel, government workers, or administrative assistants, whose careers do not depend on entertaining, but who love to eat rich meals with good wines just for the pleasure of it.

People can only keep this pattern up, however, if their livers can efficiently detoxify. Once this ability is compromised, a person will likely suffer indigestion, have severe hangovers, and suffer disturbed sleep, making entertaining more of a chore than a pleasure. Being unable to detoxify effectively can therefore limit how much a person can eat and/or drink and how often they are able to enjoy the pleasures of entertaining.

As people age, their ability to tolerate alcohol diminishes. The overconsumption of alcohol can then actually become a liability both in business and for one's health. The downsides of alcohol consumption in middle age are memory loss, weight gain, and, perhaps worst of all, the inability to act appropriately at all times.

If your job requires frequent socializing or entertaining, or if one of your great pleasures in life is enjoying rich food and drink, a preventive liver maintenance program will serve you well. To prevent the wear and tear on your liver that rich food and alcohol consumption will inevitability create, I recommend that you follow the liver restoration program discussed later on in this book.

How social and business entertaining affects women

Research studies have shown that, in general, women are markedly less able to tolerate alcohol than men. Women metabolize alcohol more slowly than men and take longer to recover from alcohol's toxic effects. Furthermore, because of women's smaller body size and higher body-fat content, alcohol tends to become more concentrated in their bodily fluids. Many of my women patients complain that after one or two drinks, they feel sleepy and often have hangovers the next day. I have noticed that I am also more susceptible to the effects of alcohol than men tend to be.

An article published in *The Female Patient Supplement* examined women's relative intolerance of alcohol and the effects that this has on their careers. The article noted that, while women do tend to drink less than men, those women who are alcohol abusers suffer greater career and social consequences.

Male alcohol abusers are treated with more sympathy than female abusers in a job setting. Women are more likely to be fired for alcohol abuse. Women are also less likely to use workplace-based rehabilitation programs. Because alcohol has a sedative and depressant effect, a significant percentage of female alcohol abusers are likely to suffer from depression, which can further hamper job performance.

The deleterious effects of alcohol are not limited simply to women's relative intolerance to this substance. An article on alcohol and the liver, published in *Gastroenterology*, stated that for women compared to men, only half as much alcohol intake resulted in a statistically significant increase in cirrhosis of the liver. The review article also presented evidence that women are more likely than men to have liver disease progress to severe liver damage.

Veronica was a successful young businesswoman working very long, hard hours in Silicon Valley. She came to see me as a patient because she found that she was drinking too much alcohol as a means to unwind and distress at the end of her long workdays. When her stress levels were higher, she was finding that she was drinking increasingly more wine or mixed drinks, just to be able to calm down in the evenings and relax enough to be able to sleep at night.

She became concerned about her dependence on drinking too much alcohol when she started to develop PMS symptoms including extreme breast tenderness and bloating which were lasting up to 10 days to two weeks each month and increased moodiness and irritability with her friends and clients. It was clear to me that the alcohol was affecting her ability to detoxify estrogen and other hormones.

In today's fast-paced business climate, women are finding themselves having the same entertaining and socializing responsibilities as men. Throughout most of this country's history, women have not been employed in positions where entertaining and socializing were a requirement of the job. Women were primarily in back-office or staff positions with little direct customer or client responsibilities.

However, this has changed completely, with many women in positions such as account executives, sales and brokers as well as upper management, with the responsibility of developing and maintaining vital business relationships. In addition, many women now own or run their own businesses and must perform all of these jobs themselves.

As with men, many women now engage in business as well as frequent social entertaining. This often means eating rich meals, consuming alcohol, getting to bed late, and then having to be up early the next day to do it all again. During my various consulting engagements, I've seen a dramatic increase in women being the focal points for entertaining. Women, because they are more sensitive to the effects of alcohol than men, may need to exercise more care in business situations where alcoholic beverages are served.

Women who work in a business and professional environment that includes socializing, need to know how to gracefully decline alcoholic drinks if they lack the ability to handle them and order a socially acceptable nonalcoholic beverage instead. Luckily, the prevalence of women professionals in virtually every career, from business to the arts and sciences, has coincided with the growing acceptance of nonalcoholic beverages such as mineral water or nonalcoholic beers. Many men are also forgoing or reducing their consumption of alcoholic beverages at professional lunches and dinners, often for health reasons but also for performance reasons.

If you do plan to indulge in alcoholic beverages and want to avoid the energy drop that can follow, the traditional concept about not drinking on an empty stomach applies. To slow down the rapid absorption of alcohol, it is important to precede its ingestion with fatty or oily foods.

Starting courses such as smoked salmon, a salad served with an oil-based dressing, or even bread and butter can prevent the liver's detoxification capability from being overwhelmed by alcohol consumed on an empty stomach. Some women may prefer to use flax-seed oil capsules, thereby gaining a health advantage as well as moderating the amount of alcohol their liver must process.

The Ability to Remain Calm Under Pressure

Peak performers in every major area of life tend to be those individuals who are able to think and strategize calmly under pressure. For example, in sports, the ability to remain calm under stress is often more important than having the physical skills to win.

Every weekend, many millions of people watching sports on television see poise, emotional control, and positive focus winning over raw talent that has lost its composure. A figure skater almost stumbles on a triple axel but rights herself and finishes the program with a flourish. A champion golfer hits the ball into a difficult lie in the deep rough but plays it out onto the green, positioned for a par-saving putt. A college basketball player sinks two free throws with almost no time left to seal a come-from-behind victory in the noisy arena of a rival.

Tennis champion Chris Evert dominated the world of women's tennis for many years even though she did not have the greatest athletic ability or foot speed. However, she was always able to play her best under the stress of competition. When she hit a bad shot or a call went against her, she was able to remain calm and in control of her thoughts and actions. She never showed anger or fear, saving all her energies and skills for winning the next point.

Although few people need to perform at the level of intensity and composure of professional athletes, many people are engaged in careers where remaining internally calm and centered during periods of stress is a prerequisite for success. Professional securities traders or emergency-room doctors and nurses are constantly making critical decisions with incomplete information under chaotic conditions. For the trader, split-second decisions to buy hold, or sell a security can mean millions of dollars in gains or losses for a client or their firm. For the emergency room doctor or nurse, the need to make rapid decisions in a crisis situation often has life-or-death consequences.

Healthy liver functioning is a physiological prerequisite for being able to remain calm and perform well under stress. Individuals with healthy detoxification function tend to be more even tempered, are more likely to demonstrate good judgment, and are better able to solve problems in a logical and impartial manner.

The deleterious effects that impaired detoxification capability has on temperament and judgment have been confirmed in a number of research studies. When liver function is impaired, toxic chemicals such as alcohol, recreational drugs, and even industrial pollutants are not properly metabolized and their toxic by-products will accumulate within the tissues of the body.

These toxic by-products can cloud judgment, affect emotional stability, and reduce the ability to perform well under stressful conditions. Individuals whose liver function is compromised are more likely to have emotional outbursts and lose their focus under duress. These people, under pressure, will tend to make poor decisions, reacting to a situation rather than calmly dealing with the issues at hand and creating effective solutions.

Many people in various walks of life limit their chances of succeeding because they have poor detox-ification function and are unable to remain calm under stress or maintain appropriate behavior. A friend of mine, Rick, found himself working briefly with such a person and shared his story with me. Bill, the manager of the project, had spent most of his career raising capital for start-up ventures in which he often took on some form of operational respon-sibility; however, a number of these projects had been mismanaged, so his performance history was inconsistent.

As Rick began to work with him, he began to understand why Bill's record was so poor. Although

Bill had an excellent education and was extremely bright and physically very strong, he had also been a heavy drinker. He had an aggressive personality, which his drinking had only worsened. When inevitable differences of opinion and communication snags arose while working on a project, Bill's response was to become overly aggressive, threaten everyone involved, and often institute legal action. Because he was unable to stay calm and find constructive solutions to problems, he routinely alienated people and developed serious interpersonal animosities.

By the time Rick started to work with him, Bill had actually quit drinking and was attending AA meetings. I met Bill on a number of social occasions, and noted that despite his discontinuance of alcohol, his diet was not supportive of healthy detoxification function. Instead of alcohol, he was continually drinking highly sugared cola drinks and coffee, snacking on chocolate chip cookies, and eating a high-fat, red meat based diet, always finishing with rich desserts. All of these foods continued to put stress on his liver, which exacerbated his belligerent and aggressive behavior. Within a year, his overly aggressive personality, abrasive behavior, and poor decisions caused him to be removed from the project.

Individuals with a history of alcohol abuse who have ceased their consumption of alcoholic beverages should also avoid using substitutes that continue to damage liver function. Soft drinks, fruit juice, tonic water, coffee or black tea, and even carbonated water should be rigorously avoided because of their high content of sugar, caffeine, and carbon dioxide (an acidic waste product of our own body's cells). All of these substances are detrimental to healthy liver function.

Instead, drink plenty of spring or filtered water or herbal teas such as peppermint and chamomile, which are traditionally used in herbal medicine to support and restore healthy liver function. In addition, highly sugared or fat-laden meals should be avoided during the period of recovery from alcohol abuse. These dietary guidelines are equally helpful for individuals recovering from other chemical addictions, such as the use of recreational drugs, or from toxic environmental exposure, since all toxic chemicals tend to compromise liver function.

I have had many patients over the years who have complained about their inability to remain calm and centered during times of stress. Often, impaired detoxification capability has played a role in causing their problem. Many of these individuals have had a history of alcohol or drug abuse. They would often describe a tendency toward overreacting to seemingly small issues with panic, upset, and even rage.

For some of these individuals, years of counseling and stress management training had not produced the desired behavioral changes. It was only when they began to treat the chemical basis of their over reactivity to stressful situations that they finally achieved mastery over their own responses. Improving the liver's ability to detoxify has been an important facet of these therapeutic programs.

If you have always been capable of operating in a calm and centered manner under stressful or adverse conditions, like the individuals described above, but have found in recent years that you are beginning to respond with less equanimity and more upset or anger, your liver's detoxification capability may be part of the problem.

These changes are often early-warning signs that your crucial detoxification function is beginning to break down, which could be due to the effects of aging or accumulated wear and tear from unhealthy lifestyle habits. In such a case, it is helpful to eliminate obvious dietary and environmental toxins and to have your detoxification capability evaluated by a health-care professional.

Summary

Good detoxification is important for anyone who wants to be at their best in the work world. It promotes a number of peak-performance traits, including physical vitality and stamina, mental clarity and acuity, the ability to get along with people, the ability to remain calm under pressure, and resistance to illness. A healthy liver also allows us to participate fully in social and business events that involve alcohol and rich foods.

5

Detoxification and Health

When the liver's ability to detoxify is weakened, blood levels of improperly metabolized chemicals begin to rise. Normally, toxins such as alcohol, drugs, environmental pollutants, and even hormones produced within the body are inactivated and broken down into harmless residues by a healthy liver.

When allowed to accumulate, however, such chemicals can be an important contributing factor to a number of diseases such as environmental allergies, chronic fatigue, alcoholic heart disease, gastrointestinal illnesses, inflammatory conditions of the nervous system, and even cancer.

The overconsumption of alcohol, fats, and refined sugar can cause hormone imbalances in both males and females, leading to elevated estrogen levels. This can increase the risk of PMS, fibroid tumors of the uterus, endometriosis, and even uterine cancer in women and abnormal breast development and alterations in sexual function in men.

Finally, the overconsumption of alcohol can lead to alcoholic hepatitis and cirrhosis of the liver, resulting in severe and permanent liver damage. Major health conditions caused by poor detoxification are discussed below.

Cold and Flu-like Symptoms

Good detoxification is a very important factor in preventing illnesses. It prevents toxic chemicals from accumulating in the body, which can cause a wide variety of distressing symptoms such as brain fog, aching joints and muscles, digestive symptoms, and even cold and flu-like symptoms.

Over the years, I have seen a number of patients develop cold and flu-like symptoms when exposed to toxic chemicals like formaldehyde, toluene, or benzene. I have also seen these symptoms in patients whose livers could not handle prescription drugs that were prescribed by their physicians for specific medical purposes. I have seen patients develop a runny nose, sneezing, and even chills when administered a local anesthetic for minor surgery.

I have even seen these types of symptoms occur after patients ingested synthetic hormones like Synthroid, a replacement therapy for low thyroid function, or Provera, a synthetic form of progesterone, as well as prednisone, an adrenal hormone used to treat many inflammatory conditions.

The cold and flu-like symptoms did not abate in these individuals until they were able to avoid exposure to the environmental toxins that they could not tolerate or until they discontinued the use of the offending drug. Symptoms often continued after minor surgery until the anesthetic was finally detoxified by the body.

Prescription drugs are not the only culprits. I have also found that very sensitive patients can occasionally even develop nausea, bloating, and other symptoms of poor liver function after taking oil-based nutritional supplements such as vitamin E, evening primrose oil, and certain herbs.

The individuals who suffer from such extreme susceptibility to environmental chemicals, medications, and nutrients are unable to detoxify them efficiently due to poor liver function. All of these substances must be broken down by the enzyme systems of the liver and then excreted from the body so as not to accumulate to toxic levels. Healthy people, whose detoxification systems are intact, tend to metabolize and excrete specific drugs at the same rate. This rate is measured as the half-life of the drug, or the amount of time required for 50 percent of it to be eliminated from the body.

Drugs with long half-lives remain in the body a longer period of time in their active form and only need to be used once a day. A drug with a shorter half-life, like aspirin, may need to be taken every four to six hours to maintain therapeutic activity. However, when an individual patient has impaired liver function, the half-life of the drug may be considerably longer, due to their inability to metabolize or excrete it. In this case, either the drug dosage may need to be revised or its use discontinued entirely.

The symptoms of colds and flus are performance and success saboteurs—making you feel miserable and often resulting in lost work time. If you frequently suffer from these symptoms, it is important to differentiate between the symptoms caused by infectious disease and reactions that are due to exposure to a toxic substance you cannot tolerate.

While colds and flus need to be treated by suppressing the pathogens and restoring your body's buffering, enzyme, and oxygenation functions, similar types of symptoms due to toxic chemical exposure need to be treated differently. Toxic chemicals need to be detoxified and eliminated from the body through healthy liver function.

Remember that cells within the liver also help to destroy disease-causing bacteria. If you are susceptible to specific drugs or nutrients, their use should be discontinued and further use avoided. However, be sure to consult with your physician before discontinuing any prescription drugs. If your symptoms seem to be due to the use of nutritional supplements, use non oil-based substitutes. In addition, you should follow a liver restoration program such as the one described in the next chapter to help restore your detoxification capability.

Chronic Fatigue and Environmental Allergies

As mentioned in this book, the exposure to a wide variety of environmental toxins can be causal factors in both chronic fatigue states and environmental allergies. When improperly detoxified, such common substances as lawn and garden pesticides and herbicides, cleaning solutions, perfumes and hair care products, and building materials can trigger allergic symptoms. These include fatigue, poor cognitive function, runny noses, eye irritation, skin rashes, headaches, nausea, joint pains, and mood changes.

If these cases of chronic fatigue and environmental sensitivity due to poor detoxification capability remain undiagnosed, the individuals affected may languish for months or years, unable to function properly at work or participate fully in their personal lives. Proper diagnosis of these conditions is mandatory. Individuals with these symptoms should seek out the help of physicians who deal with environmental illness and are knowledgeable about detoxification therapies.

Nervous System Disease

The inability of the liver to detoxify alcohol is a main cause of nervous system disease and impairment. A liver that is able to clear alcohol from the system as it is consumed acts as a protective barrier, preventing the toxic by-products of its breakdown from reaching the brain and nervous system, which are particularly vulnerable.

In chronic alcohol abuse, the liver's ability to detoxify alcohol slowly erodes over time, and there is an increase in circulating levels of alcohol in the blood. As liver disease advances, brain cells are destroyed, resulting in serious nervous system disorders, including polyneuritis (nerve inflammation), premature senility, and encephalopathy (chronic degenerative brain syndrome).

Research suggests that one possible cause of the destruction of brain cells may be an accumulation of manganese in the brain due to poor clearance by the liver. The intake of normal amounts of manganese is required for good health, but in higher amounts it can be toxic.

In a small study appearing in the *Annals of Neurology*, researchers investigated this association. The patients, aged forty-nine to sixty-five, had cirrhosis of the liver coupled with neurologic dysfunction. The researchers noted that these patients had elevated blood levels of manganese and also an accumulation of this mineral in the brain, suggesting that with impaired liver function, even normal amounts of dietary manganese can accumulate to toxic levels within the tissues.

Alcohol-Related Heart Disease

An efficiently functioning liver protects not only the brain but also the heart from being damaged by alcohol. Circulating alcohol is toxic to the heart. Alcohol decreases heart muscle action and electrical conductivity and can, over time, lead to congestive heart failure, cardiac arrhythmias, and cardiac enlargement. There is some evidence that low to moderate alcohol consumption may reduce the risk of deep venous thrombosis and pulmonary embolism in older individuals, according to a study published in the *Journal of the American Geriatric Society*.

But many studies also document the association of excess alcohol intake and potentially dangerous cardiac disease. One study, published in the *Journal of the American Medical Association*, examined the heart health of 100 asymptomatic, alcoholic men and fifty asymptomatic, alcoholic women, compared with fifty nonalcoholic women as a control group.

Of the men, 39 percent showed evidence of alcohol-related heart damage. This was found to be the case for an even higher percentage of the alcoholic women studied. In almost a third of the men, their alcohol intake was found to be a causal factor. Furthermore, women showed an even greater susceptibility to the toxic effects of alcohol as a risk factor for their disease.

Elevated Estrogen Levels

As mentioned earlier, efficient metabolism of estrogen by the liver helps to regulate hormone levels in women. Through its detoxification function, the liver helps to modulate the amount and control the type of estrogen circulating through a woman's body. Estrogen is secreted by the ovaries in a highly potent form called estradiol.

The liver metabolizes this form of estrogen so that it can be eliminated from the body, first by converting estradiol to an intermediary form called estrone and finally to a weaker form called estriol. The liver's ability to efficiently convert estradiol to estriol is important because estriol is the safest and least chemically active form of estrogen. In contrast, estrone and estradiol are very active stimulants in breast and uterine tissue.

Excessive intake of alcohol, fat, and refined sugar in females has been associated with both lack of ovulation and elevated estrogen levels. Excess estrogen can worsen the congestive symptoms of menstrual pain and cramps and cause fluid and salt retention in the body, particularly during the pre-menstrual and menstrual phases. Excess estrogen can also trigger the growth and spread of endometriosis implants, thereby worsening menstrual cramps and pain.

Overconsumption of alcohol has also been linked to heavy bleeding and spotting in women with fibroid tumors of the uterus and endometriosis. Finally, excess estrogen is a risk factor for the development of breast cancer.

Alcohol abuse also elevates estrogen levels in men. Like women, men produce estrogen, but in much smaller amounts. Normally, a healthy male secretes as much estrogen as a woman does after menopause, about 10 to 25 percent of the amount she produces during her reproductive years.

In male alcoholics, their liver may be unable to detoxify the small amount of estrogen that they produce, leading to an elevation of their blood estrogen levels. This can lead to breast enlargement and other mild symptoms of feminization. Research scientists have also observed estrogen-induced cellular changes in the prostate glands of patients with liver disease.

Sexual Problems

Many people think of alcohol as a stimulant because it reduces inhibitions and, when consumed in moderation, increases social interactions. But it is actually a sedative, suppressing emotions and potentially causing sexual issues for women and impotence in men due to its negative effect of hormone metabolism. Research studies have confirmed the negative effect that alcohol has on sexual desire and performance. This is due, in part, to hormonal imbalances caused by impaired liver detoxification.

Cancer

The development of cancer may be related to liver function, as evidenced by the link between alcohol intake and the incidence of esophageal, liver, and breast cancer. A number of recent studies suggest that drinking alcoholic beverages, even in moderate amounts, increases the risk of breast cancer.

A study conducted at the Harvard School of Public Health followed the dietary habits of 89,538 women nurses between the ages of thirty-four and fifty-nine for four years. Women who ingested between three and nine drinks per week had a 30 percent increase in their risk of breast cancer. Those who had more than nine drinks per week had a 60 percent increase.

In another research study published in *The New England Journal of Medicine*, 188 women between twenty-five and seventy-seven were followed over a ten year period. Researchers observed that the women who consumed alcohol regularly, as compared with those who did not, had a 50 percent greater risk of developing breast cancer.

When a person is undergoing chemotherapy or any cancer treatment that results in the killing of tumor cells at an accelerated rate, it is imperative that both the toxic by-products of this tumor cell destruction and the drugs themselves be quickly eliminated from the body. If these toxic chemical residues remain in the system, they can overburden the liver's detoxification capabilities and greatly increase the risk of death.

Complementary physicians usually recommend that cancer patients do everything possible to support their liver's ability to detoxify harmful substances. Liver detoxification techniques are discussed later on in this book.

6

Evaluating Your Detoxification Ability

To help you assess whether or not your body has the kind of detoxification ability that you need for good general health as well as peak performance, you can work through the following checklist. Detoxification can also be tested medically.

Checklist: Do You Have Healthy Detoxification?

Although the following checklist does not provide a definitive diagnosis of your detoxification ability, knowing what items apply to you can help determine whether your own system is working adequately. If the results of this self-quiz suggest that your liver function is weak, you may want to have laboratory testing done through your health care provider.

Put a check mark beside those statements that are true for you.

Lifestyle/Environmental Factors

- o My diet is high in sugar.
- o My diet is high in fat.
- o I tend to eat a lot of fast food.
- o I regularly consume alcohol.
- o I regularly consume caffeinated beverages, including coffee, tea, and colas.
- o I regularly consume food additives and artificial sweeteners such as aspartame.
- o I use excessive amounts of prescription drugs, over-the-counter medications, and recreational drugs.
- o I have been exposed to synthetic pesticides and herbicides.
- o I have been exposed to industrial chemicals and cleaning agents.

Performance Indicators

- o I experience brain fog upon waking in the morning.
- o I am frequently unable to think clearly and use good judgment.
- o I am often unable to remain calm under stress.
- o I have difficulty socializing and mixing easily with people because of food and alcohol intolerances.
- o I am often unable to perform tasks effectively.
- o I suffer from chronic fatigue.
- o I am often irritable.
- o I have a tendency to be impatient, arrogant, and resentful.
- o I often get angry when driving.
- o I have an explosive or impulsive personality.

Physical Indicators

- o I have vitamin and mineral deficiencies, especially the fat-soluble vitamins and vitamin B complex.
- o I have high cholesterol.
- o I have high levels of circulating estrogen.
- o I am over seventy years old.
- o I have frequent episodes of tiredness, dizziness, nausea, and a racing pulse.
- o I have a marked distaste for oily foods.
- o I experience soreness in the liver area under moderate fingertip pressure.
- o I often have poor digestion, gas pains, constipation, and a feeling of fullness in the stomach and intestines.
- o I have low levels of stomach acid and digestive enzymes.

Medical History

- o I have a history of hepatitis or other liver disease.
- o I have had a diagnosis of heart disease, such as congestive heart failure, cardiac arrhythmia, enlarged heart, or coronary heart disease.
- o I have a history of nervous-system diseases, such as polyneuritis.
- o I generally lack resistance to infectious disease.
- o I have a history of disease of the gastrointestinal tract, such as gastritis, esophagitis, pancreatitis, or ulcers.
- o I have a history of gallstones.

Laboratory Tests to Evaluate Liver Function

If you suspect your detoxification ability is impaired, you may want to consider having laboratory testing done. Traditionally, physicians have assessed liver health by ordering blood tests to measure the levels of enzymes produced by the liver, such as SGOT and SGPT. These enzymes become elevated when there is significant damage to the liver. However, newer tests are available that allow health care professionals to measure not only liver pathology but also the health of the liver's detoxification function.

Blood tests

When there is liver damage or inflammation, an elevation in the blood levels of liver enzymes can occur. Elevated levels can indicate liver damage due to exposure to toxic chemicals, excessive alcohol use, or infectious diseases such as hepatitis.

The two enzymes most commonly monitored are serum glutamic oxaloacetic transaminase (SGOT) and serum glutamic pyruvic transaminase (SGPT), which are released by liver cells when there is acute cellular destruction. Of the two enzymes, SGOT is more sensitive to cellular damage and is released even when there is only mild injury. However, SGOT is found in several types of tissue, including significant amounts in the heart, making it a less specific indicator of liver disease. SGPT requires somewhat more extensive or severe cell damage to rise above normal levels, but it is a reliable indicator of liver damage because virtually all of SGPT originates in the liver, making it a more specific test.

Detoxification profile

A detoxification profile is a relatively new procedure that tests the ability of the liver to detoxify various substances. Their metabolites are then measured in the urine, blood, or saliva. The profile measures substances that are active either in phase I or phase II of the detoxification process.

To measure the function of the phase I detoxification system, a premeasured amount of caffeine is ingested. If salivary testing is done, saliva samples are taken during the eight hours after ingestion. The caffeine's rate of clearance can be used to assess phase I detoxification activity.

To test the phase II detoxification system, individuals are given aspirin, acetaminophen, or sodium benzoate (which is used for individuals with salicylate sensitivity). The metabolites are then measured. Individuals often show great variation in their ability to detoxify, depending on the health of their liver.

Summary

Healthy liver function is essential to many aspects of peak performance as well as good general health. As we will see in the next chapter, we can support our liver's ability to detoxify our bodies in a number of ways, including dietary choices, nutritional supplementation, and several very effective liver-cleansing techniques.

Part II:
Restoring Your Ability to Detoxify

7

Introduction to my Detoxification Program

In order to maximum performance and maintain good health, the liver must be able to detoxify pollutants that the body ingests or absorbs from the environment as well as those that the body generates itself in the process of metabolism. Fortunately, there are many effective techniques that a person can use to restore their health by reestablishing the liver's ability to detoxify.

In Part II of this book, I have included a powerful three-part program to enable you to restore your detoxification ability. This program is very effective and will begin to work rapidly to help rebuild and support your liver so your detoxification capability can return to optimal functioning.

The program consists of specific dietary regimens (described in chapter 8, 9, 10) as well as the use of special liver restorative nutrients (chapter 11 and 12), which will help the liver metabolize and rid the body of toxic pollutants, chemicals, and the waste products generated by our own metabolism. I also provide you with a number of very effective liver-cleansing tech-niques (chapter 13), which will accelerate the healing of the liver as well as help it detoxify and eliminate many potentially toxic substances from the body.

Over the years, I have found that when my patients have followed a program to support liver function and enhance detoxification, they usually begin to notice a rapid reduction in their symptoms. The liver responds quickly, especially if the intake of toxic substances that burden it is significantly reduced.

A Caution on Starting Your Detoxification Program

When you are customizing your own liver detox-ification program, it is important to both cleanse the liver and strengthen and restore its functional capacity at the same time. Since powerful reactions such as headaches, fatigue, and even a runny nose can occur with any detoxification program, you must start slowly and gradually work up to suggested levels. As with all health programs, you must experiment within known safe ranges to find the levels that work for your individual biochemistry.

Pick the colon-cleansing techniques that you are most comfortable with, and use it as frequently as your occupation and lifestyle permit. As you reduce your intake of toxins like alcohol or recreational drugs, your body will begin to try to eliminate these and other toxins that have been stored at the cellular level.

The colon-cleansing techniques, in particular, will allow for the accelerated excretion of these toxins without the body having a healing crisis as the liver unloads toxins into the bloodstream and the small intestine. Colon cleanses are one of the most important things you can do while rebuilding your liver function.

8

The Detoxification Diet

Because our livers tend to get so overworked and stressed, it is important to follow a dietary program that supports the health and function of your liver and even incorporate periodic fasting. This will help to maintain your ability to detoxify efficiently. This means eliminating foods that put wear and tear on the liver and stress our bodies such as high fat and sugar laden foods, rich desserts, caffeine, alcohol, fast foods like pizza and cheeseburgers, fried foods, white flour products, and additives.

I know it can be challenging at first, but it is worth it in terms of your improved health, wellness, and better detoxification ability. It means eating a diet that is primarily composed of whole, unrefined, high nutrient foods. These foods should be organic, unsprayed, and unprocessed, whenever possible. It is essential to follow a dietary program that emphasizes lighter, easier to digest foods as well as foods that are beneficial for the liver's functioning. I discuss these dietary principles in more detail in this chapter.

I have found that when my patients have followed a diet to support healthy liver function and enhance detoxification, they usually begin to notice a rapid reduction in their physical symptoms of ill health. Their level of energy and vitality usually is increased as well as their mental clarity and sharpness. Feelings of emotional stress, like being on an "emotional roller coaster," start to smooth out. The mood becomes more calm and balanced. The liver responds quickly to a lighter, healthier diet, especially if the intake of toxic substances that burden it is significantly reduced. An added benefit is that you may find that you begin to shed unwanted pounds and that chronic health issues begin to improve.

When you are customizing your own liver detoxification program, it is important to both cleanse the liver and strengthen and restore its functional capacity at the same time. Since powerful reactions such as headaches, fatigue, and even a runny nose can occur with any detoxification program, you must start slowly and gradually work up to suggested levels. All dietary changes that are made to improve liver function should be done gradually, over several weeks to several months. As with all health programs, you must experiment within known safe ranges to find the levels that work for your individual biochemistry.

To restore the liver's detoxification capability, it is important to eat a vegetarian emphasis diet, with an emphasis on lightly steamed or raw foods. Daily meals should incorporate a variety of salads, fresh vegetables, whole grains, and legumes. These foods, which are made up of simple molecules of starch, cellulose, fruit sugars, antioxidants, and other easy-to-metabolize substances, place minimum stress on the liver.

Some people need a higher protein intake to maintain their level of energy. If animal protein is desired, small to moderate amounts of easy-to-assimilate fish, free-range poultry and eggs can be added. Oils should be high-quality cold-pressed monounsaturated and polyunsaturated vegetable oils — used only in small amounts in the early stages of recovery.

In terms of your main meal of the day, many people on a detoxification diet do well with their plate divided up between ½ vegetables or salad, ¼ complex carbohydrate-like whole grains and ¼ protein. This can vary, of course, based on your own individual dietary needs. Breakfast can includes smoothies, shakes, and nutritious whole grain cereals with ingredients like ground flax meal which benefit digestion or easily digestible protein based dishes, as needed.

More Specific Information on Diet

Traditional Chinese medicine recommends the use of certain plant-based foods as part of a dietary regimen for restoring liver function. I have found in my clinical practice that the following foods are well tolerated and seem to accelerate the healing of liver related problems: beets, broccoli, cabbage, Brussels sprouts, turnips, kale, parsley, lettuce, cucumber, green foods such as spirulina, chlorella, and barley grass, beans and peas, sprouts, tofu, rice, millet, and fruits, preferably consumed during the warmer months. However, I recommend avoiding vinegar and citrus fruits if you tend towards over acidity.

In contrast, a diet that includes large amounts of red meat, dairy products, and fatty foods burdens the liver, which must break down the large and more complex structures of these proteins and fats into triglycerides, prostaglandins, and an array of waste products that can be excreted by the body. When the liver cannot process fats, they accumulate inside liver cells, creating fatty degeneration of the liver. In time, these fats will be deposited in the arteries, leading to eventual heart problems and stroke.

As previously mentioned, to decrease stress on the liver, it is also critical to avoid certain substances, such as refined white sugar and flour, alcohol, caffeine, and drugs (other than needed prescribed medicines), because the breakdown of these products leaves toxic residues that the liver must neutralize. Following a lighter, fresher diet allows the liver to go through a gradual self-cleansing process, without causing further stress.

Eat only those foods that do not add to the stress load on the liver. Constantly experiment with the food groups suggested and find those you like and tolerate best. Incorporate these foods into recipes you enjoy or find recipes that use these food groups. Remember, it is virtually impossible to rebuild and restore liver function without eliminating foods that are high in fat and sugar content.

Individuals who are following a program to restore their detoxification capability may still want to enjoy an occasional meal of animal protein. The following suggestions will put the least strain on your liver. Eat eggs prepared simply, either soft- or hard-boiled. Avoid eggs prepared with fats and oils such as deviled or fried eggs. Choose soft-textured, easy-to-digest fish such as salmon over red meat such as pork, lamb, or beef, which are high in saturated fat and more fibrous in texture.

While you are restoring your liver function, eliminate all alcoholic beverages. Switch to mineral water and herbal teas such as chamomile and peppermint, which are therapeutic for the liver. Once liver function is restored, alcohol intake should be limited to an occasional, single beverage.

Individuals with impaired detoxification function should make an effort to avoid eating after 6:00 p.m. or 7:00 p.m. at the very latest. In addition, eat your heaviest meals early in the day, with your last meal being the lightest. This will help to prevent undue stress on the liver during the night when it should be repairing and restoring itself rather than trying to metabolize the residues of a heavy meal. Eating late at night can significantly retard a liver restoration program. Many of my patients have found that avoiding heavy meals eaten late at night significantly reduces morning grogginess and brain fog.

All dietary changes that are made to improve liver function should be done gradually, over several weeks to several months. Too extreme and rapid a change in one's diet can induce waste products to be eliminated more rapidly than the liver can handle, triggering symptoms like nasal congestion, flu-like symptoms, diarrhea, bad breath, and aches and pains.

You can continue taking any nutritional supplements that you would normally use during a modified fast in order to provide your body with the essential support that it needs.

9

Modified Fasting

Many books on detoxification recommend fasting as the most efficient and quickest way to rid the body of accumulated toxins, but true fasting is very difficult for the average American. A true fast means consuming only water or diluted liquids such as juices, broths, or herbal teas for a prescribed period of time.

Fasting has been practiced for thousands of years by the people of nearly all cultures all over the world. Used for purification, penance, during periods of mourning, and to strengthen mental, physical, and spiritual powers, fasting is an ancient practice with modern applications.

However, most of us in the United States live busy, stressful lives, with myriad responsibilities at home, school, and work. We don't often have the luxury of a large block of time without responsibilities to undertake the intensity of a true fast.

Fasting can accelerate the elimination of toxins from the body and trigger a number of uncomfortable symptoms including nasal discharge, headache and flu-like symptoms.

If you are working and active, a true fast can be very disruptive. However, I have found with my own patients that many of them do very well with a modified fasting program of two or three light meals a day.

These meals can consist of vegetable and fruit juices; low-sodium and low-fat broths; herbal teas; fresh shakes and smoothies; light, easy-to-digest solid foods, such as uncooked or lightly steamed organic vegetables and sprouts; and cooked starches, grains, and legumes. Such a program can be followed for a few days up to several weeks, although some people may choose to do this for an even longer period of time. This program will help to begin clearing toxins from the liver.

You should consume only organic vegetables during a modified fast, because if you are trying to eliminate toxins from the body, consuming foods covered with chemical pesticides and fertilizers is counter-productive. Vegetable juices should be prepared fresh, used within a day or two, and always kept refrigerated. Some bottled organic vegetable juices may be used when fresh ones are unavailable. Preferred vegetable juices are carrot, beet and beet greens, parsley, celery, cucumber, and spinach. To enhance the cleansing action of these juices, add a little garlic, ginger, or wheatgrass juice.

However, don't drink fruit juices by themselves because they are highly acidic and high in concentrated sugars. Fruit juices can be mixed with vegetable juices if you miss the sweet flavor of fruit. If you can't live without some fresh fruit juice, the best ones are papaya and melon, preferably diluted by 50 percent with water. If you are hypoglycemic or suffer from fatigue, you should avoid drinking fruit juice completely. The simple sugars found in fruit juices will cause an overproduction of insulin by the pancreas. This, in turn, will trigger the roller coaster effect of quick highs and sudden lows in blood sugar levels.

In contrast, eating the whole fruit slows down absorption of the sugar because of the fiber contained within the whole fruit. In addition, when fruit juices are mixed with protein and oils, like protein powder or ground flaxseed, the sugar from the juice is absorbed much more slowly and does not cause a hypoglycemic type of effect.

Smoothies and shakes are great meals to prepare during a detoxification diet or modified fast because they contain the full range of nutrients needed to maintain your level of energy. Yet, they do not put stress on the digestive organs, including the liver, because all of the ingredients are already broken down into small particles and liquefied in a blender, thereby making digestion much easier.

As with a detoxification diet, you can continue taking nutritional supplements that you would normally use during a modified fast in order to provide your body with the essential support that it needs.

10

Juice Fasting

If you decide that you want to try a juice fast in which you consume only fruit and vegetable juices while totally abstaining from food consumption, you will have an accelerated cleansing and detoxification of your body. Juice fasting is usually done for one to three days, although some people may choose to fast for longer period of time. However, if you choose to fast for longer periods of time, you may want to consult with your health care practitioner as to the advisability of doing this, given your particular health status.

Fasting for short periods of time can be beneficial in that it takes stress off of your digestive organs. It is particularly beneficial to the body to stop eating fast food, alcohol, coffee, soft drinks, sugar, refined flour products, fried foods, and all other foods that put excessive wear and tear on our systems.

Juice fasting can also help to accelerate weight loss and to release patterns of addiction to sugar, caffeine, soft drinks, and overeating. Some people choose to do juice fasting as part of an alternative health program to support healing from a chronic health issue or as part of a cleansing process to refresh and revitalize their bodies.

Rapid detoxification can, however, trigger several troublesome symptoms, including headaches, skin odor and/or eruptions, a displeasing taste in the mouth, a thick coating on the tongue, diarrhea and digestive upset. A person may develop flu-like symptoms or a nasal discharge for a day or two. Most people who go on a rigorous, fast experience may initially experience a drop in their energy level and have constant thoughts of food. Some people experience even more serious symptoms, such as faintness or an irregular heartbeat, which should be reported to a physician immediately.

Cautions on Juice Fasting

- If you are a pregnant or nursing woman, you should avoid juice fasting.
- If you are diabetic or suffer from severe hypoglycemia or chronic fatigue, be sure to consult with your physician about the advisability of doing juice fasting.
- If you suffer from anemia, anorexia or low body weight, kidney disease, epilepsy or other preexisting condition, I recommend that you consult with your own health care provider about the advisability of doing a juice fast.

- If you are using prescription medication I recommend that you consult with your own health care provider or physician about the advisability of doing a juice fast. Prescription medication should not be discontinued or reduced on your own.

Guidelines for Juice Fasting

When doing a fast, you should use only freshly juiced organic fruits and vegetables. Do not use commercial bottled or canned juices that are processed, as they may have been heavily sprayed with pesticides and herbicides and lack the same level of vitality as fresh juices.

Grapefruit juice should be avoided during a juice fast, especially if you are taking prescription drugs since this can affect the manner in which certain drugs are metabolized in your body.

You may want to do a modified fast, as outlined in the previous chapter, for several days up to a week before beginning and after completing a juice fast. This will help you prepare for a fast and also assist you in transitioning back to a normal diet.

Juice should be ingested throughout the day. Many people will choose to drink between 32 to 64 ounces of juice per day, but amounts can vary from person to person, depending on size and hydration needs. Be sure to drink spring or filtered water, as well, to maintain adequate hydration.

It's best to do juice fasting during the warmer months and abstain from fasting during the cold winter months when the body needs warmer, more heating foods.

Before juicing fresh fruits and vegetables, be sure to wash them thoroughly to remove any pesticides, herbicides, and dirt. Some women even wash their fruits and vegetables in a dilute solution of bleach if they are concerned about chemical contamination. Leave the skin of the fruit or vegetable intact, when possible, or pare it thinly because many nutrients are concentrated in this part of the plant. And be sure to store fresh vegetables in the refrigerator soon after obtaining them to avoid loss of nutrients.

You may continue the use of nutritional supplements that you consider to be essential for your health. However, if you are comfortable, you may want to abstain or use an abbreviated number of vitamins and minerals for a few days during the fast.

While you can continue with your normal routine during the fast, it is best to minimize or avoid doing very strenuous physical or mental activity. A daily walk is beneficial if that it promotes healthy oxygenation and circulation.

You may also find it beneficial to do cleansing techniques, including dry brush massage, colon cleansing, and enemas. This will help in the elimination of toxins from the body. I discuss these later on in the book.

Types of Juicers

There are two types of equipment that you can use to make your fresh fruits and vegetable juices: high speed blenders and juicers. I frequently make fresh juice and have worked with both types of equipment. I have found that they both make excellent quality juices, although the process and the composition of the juice can vary.

Whatever type of juicer you decide to buy, it is very important to take good care of your equipment. It should be washed and cleaned carefully after use and stored in a dark, cool area.

Blenders

Juicing fruits and vegetables in a blender liquefies the food, breaking all of its components into extremely small particles, and enhances (or replaces) the mechanical digestive step of chewing. The surface area of the food is dramatically increased, thereby eliminating one of the functions of pancreatic and other enzymes in the breakdown process and hence requiring less enzyme production.

Blenderized juice is absorbed and assimilated very easily, with minimal symptoms of incomplete or poor digestion such as bloating, gas, and food remaining in the digestive tract for long periods of time. The nutrients from the food are much more readily available when food is taken in blenderized form.

The entire fruit and vegetable, including the skin and seeds, can be liquefied in a blender thus greatly increasing the range of nutrients present in the juiced form. There is no leftover pulp with its valuable fiber that gets discarded, as with juicers. Because it processes the whole fruit and vegetable, blenderized juices can be more filling than those made by a juicer. These liquid meals can be tremendously beneficial for conditions related to either over acidity or low enzyme production such as inflammatory conditions, fatigue, brain fog, autoimmune problems, and even cancer.

Any commercially available food processor can or blender be used; however, I have found that the Vitamix (vitamix.com) super powerful blenders can pulverize virtually any whole food into a liquid very efficiently (in contrast, juicers tend to extract the juice while discarding the nutrient-rich pulp).

Juicers

There are three main types of electric juicers: centrifugal, masticating, and triturating juicers. These juicers vary by the methods that they use to extract the juice from fruits and vegetables.

Masticating – This type of juicer utilizes a single gear driven by a motor. Using this type of juicer is a slower process as it kneads and grinds fruits and vegetables that are placed in a chute. It chews up the plant fiber and breaks down the produce in a spiral rotating process. The masticating juicer is considered to be a higher quality juicer. It produces a greater quantity of juice of excellent quality.

Centrifugal – This type of juicer utilizes a spinning blade that grinds fruits and vegetables and pushes the extracted juice through a strainer. The pulp is separated from the juice so that it can be easily discarded. The juicing process occurs more rapidly than with the masticating juicer. Less juice, however, is usually extracted with a centrifugal juicer so more juice is wasted since it is retained in the pulp.

Triturating – This type of juicer utilizes twin gears and turns at a slower rpm to extract the maximum amount of juice. The process occurs in two steps. In the first step, the fruit and vegetables are crushed, while in the second step the juice is extracted. This process is thought of create a higher quality juice, despite the slowness of the process.

Nutrients Found In Fresh Fruits and Vegetables

Fresh fruits and vegetables contain a wide variety of essential nutrients that will be present in their juices, which can be of great benefit when doing a fast. In this section, I share with you some of these incredible nutrients to help you choose which fruits and vegetables you may want to include in your fast.

Benefits of Fruits

Fruits are the edible structure of flowering plants, specifically the mature ovary of the plant. (This is why when we open up a fruit we see their seeds or the offspring of the plants.) Fruits come in many shapes and colors. They delight our senses with their sweet flavors and delicious textures. Nutritionally, fruits are a treasure trove of vitamins A and C, many minerals, natural sugars, fiber, and water. Some fruits even contain protein and fat. Many studies have been done on the abundant nutrients found in fruit. Adequate fruit intake can help to prevent or relieve a wide variety of female-related health complaints, as well as many general health problems.

Fruits are an excellent source of vitamin C, which provides important protection against cancer and heart disease. In fact, vitamin C helps protect the cardiovascular system by preventing oxidation of the low-density lipoprotein cholesterol (LDL cholesterol).

This is an early event leading to the development of atherosclerosis. Certain cancers, such as cervical cancer, occur more frequently in vitamin C-deficient individuals. Vitamin C reduces capillary fragility and can help control or reduce heavy menstrual flow in susceptible women, particularly in teenage girls and in women who are transitioning into menopause.

Vitamin C also has important anti-stress and immune stimulant properties. It is needed by the adrenals for the production of adrenal cortical hormones. Women who are deficient in vitamin C due to low dietary intake or insufficient supplementation tend to handle stress less effectively, resulting in anxiety, nervous tension, and even chronic fatigue. Adequate vitamin C intake helps us to fight off a wide range of viral and bacterial infections. Vitamin C is also needed for collagen production, which maintains the structural integrity of the skin. The best fruit sources of vitamin C include citrus fruits like oranges, grapefruits, tangerines, and lemons, and other fruits such as melons, strawberries, and other berries.

Citrus fruits and berries are rich in bioflavonoids, another essential nutrient that affects blood vessel strength and permeability. Bioflavonoids also have an anti-inflammatory effect, important to women with allergies, menstrual cramps, or arthritis. Many bioflavonoids are natural sources of plant estrogens. Like our own endogenous estrogen, these weak dietary sources of estrogen can be supportive of the female reproductive tract and can improve mood and increase energy levels in women with PMS or menopausal symptoms. They can also help relieve estrogen related migraine headaches. Although citrus fruits are excellent sources of bioflavonoids and vitamin C, they are highly acidic and may be difficult to digest for some women with food allergies or sensitive digestive tracts.

Citrus fruits are used for the commercial production of bioflavonoid supplements. Unfortunately, much of the bioflavonoids in citrus fruits are found in the inner peel and pulp of the fruit. This is the bitter part of the fruit that many people discard, unaware of its health benefits. Also, the skin of grapes, cherries, and many berries are rich sources of bioflavonoids. Make sure to eat the whole fruit rather than just the juice.

Yellow and orange fruits such as cantaloupe, papaya, persimmons, apricots, and tangerines should be included in your diet because of their high vitamin A content. Vitamin A in fruit is available in high levels as a provitamin called beta-carotene. Like vitamin C, vitamin A helps to protect the body from developing many types of cancer, including cervical, lung, and bladder cancer. It also helps to protect the cardio-vascular system from heart attacks and lowers the risk of strokes.

Vitamin A in the form of beta carotene helps to improve female health in a number of other ways. Deficiencies in vitamin A have been linked to benign breast disease, heavy menstrual bleeding, and skin aging. Because it is needed for healthy mucous membranes, a lack of vitamin A can worsen the signs of aging of the vagina and genitourinary tract after menopause. Vitamin A is also essential for healthy immune function, resistance to infection, and healthy vision. Clearly, beta-carotene containing fruit should be eaten often for adequate intake of this essential nutrient.

All fruits are excellent sources of potassium, though bananas, grapefruits, berries, peaches, apricots, raisins, figs, and melons are particularly rich in this important mineral. Adequate potassium intake is necessary for good health. It helps to regulate fluid balance in the body. When women are deficient in potassium at the expense of high levels of sodium (which is ubiquitous in the American diet as table salt), health problems can occur.

Low potassium and high sodium levels can pre-dispose a person to bloating and fluid retention during the premenstrual period. In women entering menopause, a potassium deficiency can worsen fluid retention, weight gain, and high blood pressure. Women with a low potassium intake tend to tire easily and lack stamina and endurance. In fact, several studies have shown that energy levels improve significantly when a combination of potassium and magnesium supplements is taken.

Besides containing high levels of potassium, certain fruits — raisins, blackberries, and bananas, to name a few — are good sources of calcium and magnesium. You can eat these fruits often, as their minerals are essential for proper nervous system and muscular function.

In recent years, a special group of exotic fruits have been available through health food stores or through the Internet. These fruits are so rich in their antioxidant content that I call them super antioxidant fruits. These include acai berries, goji berries, noni, and mangosteen.

In case you don't know what an antioxidant is, let me explain. An antioxidant is a substance that protects our bodies from free radical damage. A free radical is a type of oxygen molecule that freely moves inside cells, reacting with proteins, fats, and DNA, changing and damaging their structure and disrupting their functions. Free radicals are generated by the metabolism of oxygen and other chemicals, including cigarette smoke, unsaturated fats, food additives, and environmental chemicals — and even by aerobic exercise. Free radicals can cause an extreme amount of damage within our bodies.

Antioxidants help to protect us from free radical damage. Antioxidants unite with free radicals and deactivate them, preventing them from doing damage. A variety of substances have an antioxidant function, including vitamin C, vitamin A, beta-carotene, vitamin E, selenium, and glutathione. It is important to either include all of the antioxidants in the diet or take them as supplements.

Super antioxidant fruits contain a high content of anthocyanins that are a subcategory of plant bioflavonoids. These are the pigments that give these fruits their strong, beautiful colors like reds and purples and are also protective antioxidants.

Super fruits like pomegranate are also a rich source of other antioxidants like polyphenols, some of which have anti-inflammatory benefits. Early research on pomegranate juice suggests that it may improve blood flow to the heart in people with coronary heart disease. It may also be beneficial in slowing the growth of prostate cancer, according to research from UCLA. There are benefits for women, too, in eating pomegranates. Pomegranates contain plant estrogens that have been found to be useful in relieving vaginal dryness.

Types of Fruits

Temperate Climate Fruits
Apples
Pears
Plums

Citrus Fruits
Grapefruit
Lemons
Limes
Oranges
Tangelos
Tangerines

Cherries
Bing
Queen Anne

Melons
Cantaloupe
Casabas
Persian honeydews
Watermelons

Grapes
Red seedless
Thompson seedless

Berries
Blackberries
Blueberries
Boysenberries
Cranberries
Gooseberries
Lingonberries
Raspberries
Strawberries

Tropical and Subtropical Fruits
Avocados
Bananas
Coconut
Guavas
Kiwis
Papayas
Pineapples

Super Antioxidant Fruits
Acai berry
Goji berry
Mangosteen
Noni Berry
Pomegranate

Benefits of Vegetables

The term "vegetables" refers to any herbaceous plant that can be eaten whole or in part. This can include the tubers, roots, stems, leaves, seeds, and flowering parts of the plant. These excellent foods come in a multitude of flavors, colors, and textures. They are composed primarily of water and carbohydrates and contain little protein or fat. They are also rich sources of many essential vitamins and minerals and provide needed bulk and fiber to the diet.

In the past few decades, many studies have concluded that the nutrients found in vegetables play an important role in protecting us from health problems. These essential nutrients include vitamin A, vitamin C, calcium, magnesium, potassium, iron, iodine, and more. In addition, vegetables contain other chemicals that help protect against heart attacks and boost immune function.

The form of vitamin A found in foods is beta-carotene, a provitamin, which is converted to vitamin A once it's taken into the body through the diet by the liver and intestines. Beta carotene is found in high doses in fruits and vegetables and is quite safe. For example, one glass of carrot juice or a sweet potato, each contain 20,000 IU of beta carotene. Many people eat two to three times this amount in their daily diet. In contrast, high doses of supplemental vitamin A derived from fish liver oil can accumulate in the liver to toxic levels.

Good sources of beta-carotene include squash, sweet potatoes, peppers, carrots, kale, spinach, turnip greens, collards, green onions, and romaine lettuce, among others. You should eat these foods often because research demonstrates that vitamin A can protect against cancer and immune problems. In women who are prone to allergies and infections, sufficient vitamin A intake can help bolster immune protection by strengthening the cell walls and mucous membranes. This protects against developing respiratory disease, as well as allergic episodes. In addition, research has linked low vitamin A levels to breast cancer, cervical cancer, bladder cancer, prostate cancer, lung cancer, and benign breast disease.

Vitamin A can play an important role in maintaining the health of women during their menopausal transition and postmenopausal years. One study from the University of South Africa found that women with heavy menstrual bleeding (a common problem as women transition into menopause) had lower blood vitamin A levels than normal volunteers.

Other studies suggest that a high intake of beta carotene containing foods protects against heart attacks in high-risk people. *The Nurse's Health Study*, sponsored by Harvard University Medical School found that women consuming 15 to 20 mg per day of beta-carotene had a 40 percent lower risk of strokes and a 22 percent lower risk of heart attacks when compared to women consuming less than 6 mg per day. Vitamin A deficiency has also been linked to fatigue, night blindness, skin aging, loss of smell, loss of appetite, and softening of bones and teeth.

Many vegetables are also high in vitamin C. These include Brussels sprouts, broccoli, cauliflower, kale, peppers, parsley, peas, and tomatoes. Vitamin C helps to strengthen capillaries and prevent capillary fragility, thereby facilitating the flow of essential nutrients throughout the body and the excretion of waste products out of the body.

This is especially important for women transitioning into menopause who are prone to heavy menstrual bleeding. When used in combination with bioflav-onoid-containing foods like soy, alfalfa, and buck-wheat, foods high in vitamin C can actually help decrease menstrual flow.

Vitamin C is also an important anti-stress vitamin because it is needed for healthy adrenal hormone production (the adrenal glands help us deal with stress). This is particularly important for women with anxiety due to emotional causes, allergies, or stress from other origins. Vitamin C is valuable for immune function and wound healing. Its anti-infectious properties may help to reduce the tendency toward respiratory, bladder, and vaginal infections. Research also suggests that along with vitamin A, vitamin C may help protect women from developing cervical cancer.

Vegetables are also outstanding foods for their high mineral content. Many vegetables are high in magnesium calcium, potassium, and which help to relieve and prevent the symptoms of menstrual cramps and PMS. Besides helping to relax tense muscles, these minerals also calm the emotions. Both calcium and magnesium act as natural tranquilizers, a benefit for women suffering from menstrual pain, discomfort, and irritability. Potassium assists in relieving the symptoms of premenstrual bloating by reducing fluid retention. These minerals are found in abundance in bone and help to provide strength to our bones. They also help to regulate the electrical activity of the heart and provide alkalinity to the body.

As you can see, calcium, magnesium and potassium are very important minerals for the overall health of our bodies. Some of the best sources for these minerals include Swiss chard, spinach, broccoli, beet greens, mustard greens, sweet potatoes, kale, green beans potatoes and peas. These vegetables are also high in iron, which may also help to reduce cramps. In addition, the calcium, magnesium, potassium, and iron found in vegetables also help protect against the development of anemia, osteoporosis, and excessive menstrual bleeding.

These minerals can also increase and maintain energy levels. Calcium, magnesium, and potassium help to improve stamina, endurance, and vitality. Clinical studies have shown that supplemental magnesium and potassium reduce depression and increase energy levels dramatically. Iodine and trace minerals are essential for healthy thyroid function and thus, maintaining a steady energy level; vegetables like kelp and other types of seaweed are high in these minerals.

Vegetables contain not only high levels of vitamins and minerals, but also other chemicals that help prevent heart attacks and boost immune function. Onions and garlic decrease blood clotting and lower serum cholesterol, which can de-crease the incidence of stroke and heart attack. Garlic has also been found to prevent and slow tumor growths in animals. Studies indicate that ginger root, onions, and mushrooms may have a similar effect. Certain mushrooms may even stimulate immune function.

Vegetables like broccoli and cauliflower contain chemicals called indoles and isothiocyanates, which help block the activation of carcinogens, such as tobacco smoke, before they cause harm to the body.

Green leafy vegetables like spinach, kale, and collard greens contain essential antioxidants like lutein and zeaxanthin, which reduce your risk of macular degeneration. Lutein is necessary healthy ovulation and progesterone production in women thereby helping to reduce estrogen dominance in the pre-menopause transition. It also reduces the risk of cardiovascular disease. I usually eat a serving of green leafy vegetables every single day for their health benefits!

Vegetable Groups

Root Vegetables
Beets
Carrots
Garlic
Onions
Radishes
Rutabagas
Turnips

Cruciferous Vegetables
Broccoli
Brussels sprouts
Cabbage
Cauliflower

Gourds
Acorn squash
Butternut squash
Chayote
Crook-neck
Squash
Cucumber
Pumpkin
Zucchini squash

Nightshades
Chili pepper
Eggplant
Garden pepper
Paprika
Potatoes
Sweet potatoes
Tomatoes

Leafy Greens
Chard
Kale
Lettuce
Collard greens
Spinach
Dandelion greens

Mushrooms
Button
Shiitake

11

Nutritional Supplements to Restore Detoxification

There are many nutrients that help to repair the liver, maintain optimal liver function and detoxification. These include antioxidants such as lecithin, vitamins C and E, the B complex vitamins, amino acids, and essential fatty acids. In liver disease, poor nutritional status is common. The following section discusses in detail those nutrients especially important to the numerous chemical reactions that make up the detoxification process.

Antioxidants

The health of the liver depends on having sufficient levels of antioxidants in the liver tissue to scavenge free radicals that interfere with liver functioning. A free radical is a type of oxygen molecule that freely moves inside cells, reacting with proteins, fats, and DNA, changing their structure and disrupting their functions.

Free radicals are generated by the metabolism of oxygen and other chemicals, including unsaturated fats, cigarette smoke, environmental chemicals, and food additives, — and even by aerobic exercise. It is estimated that about 17 percent of our total oxygen consumption turns into free radicals.

The process of detoxification itself also generates a certain amount of free radicals as by-products of the chemical reactions involved, and an accelerated detoxification process, such as that which occurs during a modified fast or cleansing program, will generate even higher levels of free radicals than normal.

Antioxidants unite with free radicals and deactivate them, preventing them from doing damage. A variety of substances have an antioxidant function, including vitamin C, beta-carotene, vitamin E, selenium, and glutathione. It is important to either include all of the antioxidants in the diet or take them as supplements. Selenium, for example, increases the effectiveness of vitamin E.

A study in the *Journal of Hepatology* found low levels of selenium in both alcoholic and nonalcoholic liver disease. The liver itself produces two important antioxidant enzymes, superoxide dismutase (SOD) and glutathione peroxidase (GP). Because these antioxidant enzymes are unstable and cannot be supplemented, it is especially important to maintain their production and function.

Both human and animal studies document a variety of ways in which antioxidants support liver health. In a paper published in the *Journal of the American College of Nutrition*, thirteen healthy males were given supplemental ascorbic acid (vitamin C) along with alcohol. The vitamin C allowed the liver to clear the alcohol more easily by accelerating its breakdown. In addition, vitamin E has been shown to have a protective effect on the liver after exposure to carbon tetrachloride, a known liver toxin.

Suggested Dosage for Vitamin E: 400 to 1200 IU (International Units) per day, preferably taken in the d-alpha-tocopherol form. While vitamin E rarely causes side effects, occasional cases have been reported of an elevation in blood pressure in individuals with preexisting hypertension. Vitamin E might also affect insulin requirements in diabetics.

In both of these cases, it is best to err on the side of caution and begin taking vitamin E at lower dosages, preferably 100 IU, and increase gradually, monitoring either blood pressure or blood sugar levels as needed. I have rarely seen any problems arising from vitamin E use; probably fewer than ten patients out of the many thousands I have worked with have had problems.

These few patients reported minor side effects like digestive upsets and skin rashes using vitamin E.

Given the millions of people who take vitamin E in this country and rarely report any unpleasant side effects, it is a remarkably safe nutrient for the vast majority of people.

Note: Use natural vitamin E instead of the synthetic form. Research studies have primarily used natural vitamin E derived from wheat germ oil. To tell the difference, read the label on the bottle. Natural vitamin E is listed as d-alpha while the synthetic is listed as dl-alpha. Although the synthetic form is less expensive, there is some concern that it is also less effective.

Suggested Dosage for Vitamin C: 1 to 5 g of mineral buffered vitamin C per day, in divided doses. Because vitamin C is water-soluble and is quickly excreted, for maximum benefit, you must take this vitamin several times during the day. Individuals who are overly acidic should use buffered vitamin C. Vitamin C is not toxic in large doses, but taking more than the body needs will cause diarrhea, a reliable sign of overdose.

Suggested Dosage for Beta-Carotene: 25,000 to 75,000 IU per day. Beta-carotene in standard dosages is not toxic. Symptoms of toxicity include nausea, enlargement of the liver and spleen, blurred vision, and skin rashes. In extremely rare cases, high doses color the skin orange. Symptoms disappear in a few days if the vitamin is withdrawn.

Special Antioxidants

D-Glucarate

Glucuronidation, a detoxification process that occurs in the liver, depends on glucuronic acid, a chemical produced within the body which is similar to calcium d-glucarate, a naturally occurring substance found in many fruits and vegetables. As estrogen circulates through the blood, it passes through the liver, where it is bound to glucuronic acid. This binding process inactivates the estrogen, inhibiting it from binding to tissues. It is then secreted into the bile and passed into the intestinal tract, where it is then eliminated from the body via bowel movements.

Unfortunately, certain bacteria in the intestinal tract secrete an enzyme called beta-glucuronidase (B-glucuronidase) which can sabotage the glucuron-idation process. B-glucuronidase breaks the newly formed estrogen-glucuronic acid bond apart, which reactivates the estrogen. This free estrogen can then be reabsorbed from the digestive tract back into the circulation, thus elevating the level of estrogen circulating through the body.

Luckily, eating a diet rich in glucarate or using glucarate supplements helps to decrease the level of

B-glucuronidase by allowing the bond between glucuronic acid and estrogen to be maintained so the body can rid itself of excess estrogen. This helps to prevent your own level of estrogen from rising to toxic levels.

D-glucarate rich foods include apples, apricots, broccoli, brussels sprouts, cherries and lettuce.

Suggested Dosage: To reduce the total amount of circulating estrogen, I also recommend taking 500 to 1,000 mg of glucarate per day with meals. This supplement is very well tolerated with no toxicity or known drug interactions.

Limonene

Another ally to help lower your total estrogen load is limonene, a compound usually found in citrus fruits, especially lemons and oranges. In addition to supporting glucuronidation, limonene also promotes healthy detoxification. Specifically, it has been shown to help prevent the development of estrogen-dependent breast cancer by stimulating detoxification enzymes in the liver.

A study published in *Cancer Research* tested to see if limonene could reduce or regress breast cancer in rats. Researchers fed a limonene-rich diet to rats that had developed breast tumors. They found that the rats that were given this diet had significant tumor shrinkage as compared to the control group. However, when the limonene was discontinued, the tumors reappeared. Additionally, researchers found that limonene inhibited the spread or metastasis of the cancer.

Limonene-rich foods include caraway, cherries, dill, lemons, oranges, mint and tomatoes.

Suggested Dosage: To help reduce free-floating estrogen in your body, I also recommend taking 500–1,000 mg of limonene per day or every other day.

Note: Women who are allergic to citrus should not take limonene. Additionally, while it appears to be safe and without toxicity, women who are pregnant or nursing should not take limonene since no research has been performed that specifically examines its effect on fetal development.

Eat a wide variety of antioxidant rich foods for optimal health. The research on breast disease, both benign and cancer, as well as osteoporosis demonstrates the benefits of including a wide variety of high antioxidant content foods in your diet. Nearly 30 percent of American women suffer from fibro-cystic breasts. And, it's no surprise that the standard American diet is partly to blame. Researchers have found that caffeine (coffee, black tea, cola, and chocolate), as well as excessive saturated fat and salt play a large role in the disease. Fortunately, by reducing or eliminating these foods from your diet and eating foods high in fiber, lots of antioxidant rich fresh fruits and vegetables, raw seeds and nuts, and flaxseeds and wild-caught seafood, you can reduce your risk for fibrocystic breasts.

DIM

DIM, or diindolylmethane, is a plant-compound found in brassica veggies such as broccoli, bok choy, cauliflower, cabbage, and Brussels sprouts. Researchers have found that this interesting little compound is quite beneficial in promoting healthy estrogen metabolism in the liver.

During estrogen metabolism, the most potent form of estrogen (estradiol) is converted into estrone. Estrone then becomes either 2-hydroxyestrone (a "good" estrone metabolite) or 16-alpha-hydroxyestrone (a "bad" estrogen metabolite). The good metabolite is then converted into 2-methoxyestrone and 2-methoxyestrodial.

This is where DIM comes in. Research has shown that when DIM is ingested, it not only encourages its own metabolism, but that of estrogen. While it is not an estrogen or even an estrogen-mimic, its metabolic pathway exactly coincides with the metabolic pathway of estrogen. When these pathways intersect, DIM favorably adjusts the estrogen metabolic pathways by simultaneously increasing the good estrogen metabolites and decreasing the bad 16-alpha-hydroxyestrone.

The research confirms this action. In a study from *Epidemiology*, American researchers took urine samples from 34 healthy postmenopausal women. They then added 10 grams of broccoli a day to the women's diets. After taking another urine sample, researchers found that this dietary change signify-cantly increased the 2-hydroxyestrone to 16-alpha-hydroxyestrone ratio.

Suggested Dosage: Make sure you are getting plenty of this amazing antioxidant by loading up on broccoli, bok choy, kale, cauliflower, cabbage, and brussels sprouts. In addition to eating more brassica vegetables, I recommend taking 30 mg of DIM a day with meals.

B Complex Vitamins

The vitamin B complex includes thiamine (B1), riboflavin (B2), niacin (B3), pantothenic acid (B5), vitamin B6, vitamin B12, folic acid, biotin, choline, and inositol. They are water soluble and are not stored well in the body, requiring that some be consumed each day, in food or supplements. People who eat a diet of mostly processed foods high in white sugar and flour, as well as those who consume a lot of alcohol, need greater amounts of B complex vitamins.

The richest source of B vitamins is brewer's yeast, but other good sources include the germ and bran of cereal grains and animal liver. Some B vitamins are also made in the intestines. Antibiotics such as sulfa drugs and tetracycline can interfere with this production, so when taking medications such as these, it is important to supplement your diet. B vitamins are critical for the production of energy within the cells and are also vital for the metabolism of fats.

The B vitamins play several roles in maintaining the health of the liver. They are necessary for the deactivation of excess estrogen, which was initially documented in studies by Morton S. Biskind in the early 1940s. Thiamine is needed for the metabolism of alcohol to degrade it to nontoxic carbon dioxide and water. Animal studies indicate that niacin protects against carbon tetrachloride poisoning and lowers cholesterol and triglyceride levels in the blood. And folic acid and vitamin B12 have been shown to counteract fatty liver (accumulation of fat within the liver).

Vitamin B deficiencies are common factors in most liver diseases. The treatment of alcoholic liver disease, for example, requires supplementation with thiamine, vitamin B6, and folic acid. Macrocytic anemia, which is associated with liver disease, requires folic acid and vitamin B12.

Suggested Dosage: A standard dose for most B-complex nutritional supplements is between 25 and 100 mg per day. (However, some of the nutrients contained within these products, like folic acid, biotin, and B12, are included in smaller amounts, measured in micrograms.)

Lecithin

Lecithin is made up of two B-complex vitamins: choline and inositol. It is a main building block of cell membranes, making up 65 percent of the membranes of liver cells. Consequently, it is one of the most important nutrients for the liver. Metabolism of various pollutants, alcohol, viruses, drugs, and other toxins occurs on the surface of cell membranes, and in this process, the detoxification enzymes produce reactive metabolites that attack liver tissue.

According to an article published in *The Alternative Medicine Review*, two decades of clinical trials provide evidence that supplemental lecithin speeds the regeneration of damaged tissue. Lecithin is used in the treatment of hepatitis, fatty liver, and alcoholic liver disease.

Lecithin also helps to prevent atherosclerosis by inhibiting low-density lipoproteins from interacting with arterial receptors, according to a study published in *Atherosclerosis*. Good sources of lecithin are egg yolks, brewer's yeast, wheat germ, fish, peanuts, leafy green vegetables, and animal liver.

The components of lecithin, choline and inositol, are classified as lipotropic factors (substances that help prevent the accumulation of fat in the liver), and as components of bile, which accelerates fat excretion. Choline is a very sensitive compound, easily destroyed by alcohol, estrogen, sulfa drugs, and cooking.

In a double-blind study published in *Liver*, choline was given for three days to fifteen patients with chronic active hepatitis. A significant reduction in disease activity was noted in patients receiving the choline. The body has large stores of inositol, which is found in whole grains, citrus, and unrefined molasses, and is depleted by drinking coffee.

Suggested Dosage: To supplement your diet with lecithin, take 2 tbsp. stirred into 4 oz. of water, once a day. The range of dosage for both choline and inositol is 50 to 500 mg. You can also add lecithin to hot cereal.

Amino Acids

While many people take vitamins and minerals, supplementing with amino acids, the building blocks of protein, is less common. Nonetheless, certain amino acids, such as methionine, glutathione, cysteine and other amino acids aid in the process of detoxification and can be taken as nutritional supplements. They are generally available in natural-food stores as well as certain pharmacies.

Methionine

Methionine is an essential amino acid, which means that it cannot be made within the body and must be supplemented or supplied by the diet. Good dietary sources of methionine include beef, chicken, beans, eggs, yogurt, onions, and garlic. It is one of the sulfur containing amino acids and is a powerful detoxifier with a long list of functions. For example, methionine can rid the body of heavy metals such as lead and mercury. It functions as an antioxidant, scavenging free radicals generated by the breakdown of toxins such as alcohol.

Methionine promotes the production of lecithin, this is required in the breakdown of fats, preventing accumulation of fat in the liver. If it is unchecked, fatty accumulation can lead to cirrhosis of the liver. Many human and animal studies show abnormalities in methionine pathways as one cause of this disease. Methionine also maintains the body's reserves of glutathione peroxidase, the powerful anti-oxidant enzyme.

Suggested Dosage: Dosages for methionine used for detoxification range from 200 to 1000 mg per day. The supplement has a meaty, sulfurous odor. It tends to be packaged in 100 to 500 mg capsules. Unfortunately, methionine is normally converted within the body to a substance called homocysteine, which is toxic to the heart. To prevent the buildup of homocysteine, 25 to 50 mg of vitamin B6 should be taken with methionine. However, rather than using methionine, I recommend instead supplementing with cysteine or n-acetyl cysteine which are produced from methionine but are safer to use. They are also discussed in this chapter.

Glutathione

Glutathione is an extremely important amino acid in the detoxification process. It is a compound amino acid composed of cysteine, glutamic acid, and glycine. It is used by complementary medical practitioners for the prevention and treatment of a variety of degenerative conditions associated with the aging process.

Like vitamins A, C, and E, glutathione is a deactivator of free radicals in the body and assists in slowing the cross-linking of collagen fibers. Cross-linking of protein fibers is a characteristic sign of aging in which the tissues become constricted and tight. It is most noticeable in older persons whose skin has taken on a leathery characteristic. However, that is just the external deterioration; cross-linking is going on throughout the entire body.

Studies have shown that glutathione also acts as an immune system enhancer and assists the body in removing heavy metals such as mercury, lead, and aluminum. Glutathione is especially important for the liver in that it helps prevent damage from alcohol by assisting in the detoxification of liver per-oxidation. Through the action of glutathione-S-trans-ferase, the liver can break down toxins into substrates for excretion via bile into the small intestine.

Glutathione is available through eating fresh fruits and vegetables, fish, and meat. Supplementary oral glutathione can be purchased in health food stores; however, it is not particularly well absorbed when taken orally. In addition, 500 to 2000 mg of vitamin C per day can elevate glutathione levels within the body by helping the body to manufacture it.

Suggested Dosage: 1000 to 2000 mg per day.

Cysteine

Methionine gives rise to the amino acid cysteine, the precursor to glutathione, which the body uses to synthesize glutathione, peroxidase and reductase, the detoxification enzymes. These antioxidant enzymes prevent the oxidation of fats and help break down toxins from car exhaust, smoke, drugs, radiation, and other carcinogens. In a study conducted in Ghana, published in *The Journal of International Medical Research*, researchers concluded that low levels of cysteine and glutathione may increase the risk of liver toxicity from oxidants.

Suggested Dosage: The dosage of cysteine is 200 mg twice a day, taken with meals. Cysteine should be taken in conjunction with 50 mg of vitamin B6 three times per day and with supplemental vitamin C (ascorbic acid) to prevent kidney stones.

N-Acetyl Cysteine (NAC)

Body levels of glutathione can also be increased by supplementing with N-acetyl cysteine (NAC), which converts to glutathione once inside the cells. NAC is more beneficial as a supplement than glutathione itself, which is not well absorbed. Not only does NAC boost our detoxification capability, but it improves immune function as well. Research studies have found that it can reduce flu symptoms when 600 mg are taken twice a day.

Suggested Dosage: A standard dosage is 300 to 600 mg once or twice per day.

Glycine and Taurine

Glycine is an essential part of glutathione, along with cysteine and glutamic acid. Thus, it plays an important role in healthy detoxification. Along with taurine, glycine conjugates or binds with bile acids to maintain the solubility of fats and cholesterol in bile, thereby helping to prevent the formation of gallstones. (Bile is a substance secreted by the liver which is stored in the gallbladder and then secreted into the small intestine.) Bile has an emulsifying effect on the fat contained in food.

Suggested Dosage: Take glycine and taurine together on an empty stomach. A standard dosage is 500 mg of glycine and 1000–3000 mg taurine per day.

Essential Fatty Acids

Because the liver is prone to inflammatory disease and all toxins cause an inflammatory reaction, it is important to consume certain oils that counteract the inflammatory response. These are the omega-3 fatty acid oils, like flaxseed oil, which have a high percentage of alpha linolenic acid and are beneficial to liver health. Eicosapentaenoic acid (EPA) and docosahexaenoic acid (DHA), found in omega-3 fatty acid rich fish like salmon, mackerel, trout, and tuna, are also beneficial for liver health. In contrast, excessive consumption of saturated fats such as those found in red meat, dairy products, and palm kernel oil promotes inflammation.

The omega-3 and the omega-6 fatty acids found in plant oils such as sesame and sunflower make up the cell walls of the mast cells, which are distributed throughout the body. These cells protect us against viruses, bacteria, and allergens by releasing material that is toxic to these invaders.

When there are sufficient omega-3s in the diet, the structure of the mast cell walls is stable, but when there is a predominance of omega-6s, the cell walls can break down more readily, releasing the fatty acids. These fatty acids enter the general circulation and are eventually metabolized by the liver. Within the liver, their chemical structure is altered, both desaturating and elongating the fatty acids.

As the omega-6 fatty acids are metabolized, they may enter the arachidonic cascade, which is a series of chemical reactions that generate primarily arachidonic acid and secondarily series II prostaglandins and leukotrienes. These are hormone-like substances that can trigger an inflammatory response and impair liver function. Studies have shown that the production of leukotrienes increases the risk of inflammatory liver diseases. Red meat and dairy foods also contain arachidonic acid, and these foods as well can lead to inflammation.

In contrast, the breakdown of omega-3 fatty acids does not enter the arachidonic pathway and therefore does not trigger the same inflammatory reactions. The omega-3 fatty acids are actually anti-inflammatory in their effects on the body.

To promote healthy liver function and prevent inflammation, there should be a balance of these fats and oils in the diet. While omega-6 fatty acids and the saturated fats found in red meat and dairy products need to be consumed judiciously, they should not be avoided completely. In fact, the omega-6 fatty acids contribute to the health of the liver in ways unrelated to their participation in the inflammatory pathways.

A study in *Alcohol and Alcoholism* found evening primrose oil, which contains high amounts of omega-6 fatty acids, to be effective in preventing liver damage caused by alcohol and in reducing alcohol withdrawal symptoms. However, as many as eight to thirteen capsules of evening primrose oil must be taken on a daily basis to attain therapeutic levels. A more practical option is to use borage seed oil, which contains a more concentrated form of beneficial fatty acids. Two to four capsules per day of borage seed oil is sufficient to reach therapeutic levels.

It is important to buy oils that are unrefined and cold-pressed to avoid the toxic by-products that occur in processed oils during the extraction process. Flaxseed oil is delicate and requires special handling. As it breaks down quickly when exposed to light, oxygen, and heat, it should never be used for cooking but only added to foods just before eating them. Flaxseed oil is usually sold in small quantities in an opaque container, found in the refrigerator section of natural-food stores. The date at which the oil was processed is found on the container, and the oil should be used only during the time specified.

Suggested Dosage: To supplement your intake of essential fatty acid, take 1 to 2 tbsp. of flaxseed oil a day and 2000-3000 mg per day of EPA and DHA in combination. Good supplemental sources of omega-6 fatty acids are evening primrose oil, eight to thirteen capsules per day, or two to four capsules of borage oil per day.

Individuals with poor liver function should begin fatty-acid therapy in very small amounts. Use one-quarter to one-third the recommended dose and increase gradually to therapeutic levels. People with poor liver function may find that fatty-acid use may initially cause nausea, abdominal bloating, and even diarrhea.

In such cases, an accelerated liver-cleansing program (discussed later in this book) and more readily tolerated liver restorative nutrients such as lecithin and antioxidants should be instituted for several months before starting fatty-acid therapy.

Whole flaxseeds, ground up in a blender or food processor or bought prepackaged in health food stores can be used stirred into cereal or in shakes. This can provide an excellent alternative to the use of flaxseed oil.

Besides their high oil content, flaxseeds are extremely rich in a wide variety of nutrients that are beneficial for the entire body, as well as the liver. Ground flaxseeds contain the entire range of essential amino acids in an easy-to-assimilate form as well as large amounts of valuable alkaline minerals such as zinc calcium, potassium and magnesium. They are an excellent source of fiber, mucilage, and lubricants, which promote the excretion of fats and other waste products from the body, thereby reducing the load on the liver. Organically grown flaxseeds are available at most health food stores and fairly inexpensive. I have developed the following flaxseed recipes that can used for breakfast or a snack.

Flax Shake No. 1   **Serves 1**

2 - 4 tablespoons ground raw flaxseeds
½ ripe papaya
1 - 1½ cups nondairy milk
Rice bran syrup, cinnamon, or nutmeg, can be added
if desired

Combine all the ingredients in a blender or food
processor and run it on high speed for 60 to 90
seconds or until the drink is totally liquefied. Add
more water if a thinner drink is desired. Drink
immediately.

Flax Shake No. 2   Serves 1

2 - 4 tablespoons ground raw flaxseeds
1 ripe banana
1 - 1½ cups nondairy milk
Rice bran syrup, cinnamon, or nutmeg, can be added if desired

Combine all the ingredients in a blender or food processor and run it on high speed for 60 to 90 seconds or until the drink is totally liquefied. Add more nondairy milk if a thinner drink is desired. Drink immediately.

Instant Flax Cereal   Serves 1

4 tablespoons raw ground flaxseeds
⅔ cup soy or other nondairy milk
½ ripe banana, sliced
Rice bran syrup, cinnamon, or nutmeg, can be added
if desired

Place the ground flaxseeds in a cereal bowl and slowly add the nondairy milk, stirring until the mixture thickens to a texture similar to that of cream of rice or oatmeal. Top the cereal with the sliced banana. Add sweetener and eat right away.

12

Herbs and Green Foods for Healthy Detoxification

The following herbs are proven tonics for the liver. They have a wide range of therapeutic benefits. Many herbs increase the flow of bile from the liver. They also stimulate increased blood flow through the liver, removing debris, old cells, and toxins. These herbs also protect the liver from a wide variety of everyday environmental toxins, such as cleaning agents and cigarette smoke, and encourage the production of enzymes that facilitate detoxification. Some of these herbs stimulate the growth of new liver cells when there is damage to the liver.

I recommend that the herbs discussed in this section be taken primarily as capsules or as teas (if palatable). I do not advise the use of tinctures and extracts for my patients with liver conditions or for those who are attempting to restore liver function, if the tinctures and extracts are processed with, and preserved in, alcohol. Alcohol, of course, adds to the toxic load of the liver and should be avoided when using herbs for liver restoration.

Silymarin

Milk thistle plant has been used for centuries as an herbal medicine. A group of the most potent and medicinally active flavonoids found in the seed of the milk thistle plant are known collectively as silymarin. In Europe, silymarin has long been prescribed for both acute and chronic liver disease. Its effectiveness has been confirmed by more than 300 studies.

Silymarin is used to treat jaundice, hepatitis, fatty liver, cirrhosis, and congestion of the bile ducts, as well as disorders of the spleen, gallbladder, and digestive tract. In a double-blind study published in the *Scandinavian Journal of Gastroenterology*, forty-seven patients, primarily with alcohol-induced liver disease, showed significant improvement with silymarin treatment. This was evidenced by a reduction in the enzymes SGPT and SGOT, which become elevated when the liver is damaged.

Silymarin protects the liver from environmental pollutants, including smoke from tobacco, coal, oil, and incense; X-rays and the side effects of radiation therapy; and industrial toxins including carbon tetrachloride. Animal studies demonstrate silymarin's action to be comparable to that of penicillin in counteracting poisons. There is some documentation of silymarin's ability to protect against nonmelanoma skin cancer and leukemia. Studies indicate that silymarin functions as a powerful antioxidant, scavenging free radicals that can damage liver cells. It also inhibits depletion of glutathione, one of the liver's most important antioxidant enzymes.

When liver cells are damaged by poisons, silymarin accelerates the rate of regeneration and protein synthesis of liver cells. It prevents the reabsorption of poisons once they leave the liver and pass through the gastrointestinal tract. This reduces the toxic load on the liver and spares the cells not yet poisoned so that they can act as centers for the generation of new liver cells. With time, complete restoration of the liver is possible.

Suggested Dosage: Milk thistle extract is considered completely safe to take in normally prescribed amounts. However, some people may experience loose stools during the first few days of taking this herb. Products containing milk thistle extract in combination with other liver restorative herbs are also available. Milk thistle extract is combined in these products with herbs such as turmeric, artichoke leaf, dandelion, or licorice. Milk thistle extract standardized to 80 percent silymarin is available in 150 to 175 mg capsules. Take one to three capsules per day.

Dandelion

Dandelion, which can grow rampant in your lawn, is a low-growing perennial plant used medicinally for over a thousand years. Arab physicians in the tenth century prescribed dandelion as a diuretic, and by the seventeenth century the English herbalist Nicholas Culpepper incorporated dandelion as the foundation of many medicinal remedies. The early English colonists introduced dandelion to North America, where it grows in many regions of the continent.

Dandelion is often prescribed to help detoxify the liver and also to prevent gallstones. Dandelion increases the flow of bile from the liver, facilitating the detoxification process. This is supported by German research, and German physicians routinely prescribe dandelion to prevent gallstones. Herbalists also often use dandelion, because of its diuretic properties, in the treatment of conditions involving fluid retention, such as PMS, obesity, high blood pressure, and congestive heart failure. As a diuretic, dandelion helps eliminate toxins from the body via the urine. It is also high in easily assimilated minerals, adding to its benefits.

Suggested Dosage: Dandelion is included in the FDA's list of herbs generally regarded as safe. In sensitive individuals, dandelion may cause a skin rash. It should not be used by women who are pregnant or nursing. When used as a food, dandelion leaves can be enjoyed in a salad. Mixed with other greens, they lend a slightly bitter sharpness. The leaves can also be taken as an infusion. Make a tea using 1/2 oz. of dried leaves per one cup of boiling water and steep ten minutes, drinking a maximum of three cups a day. Dandelion is also available in 150 mg capsules. Take one to three capsules per day.

Artichoke

The artichoke is a thistle-like plant that actually belongs to the daisy family. It is prescribed extensively in Europe to protect against toxins and to encourage the regeneration of liver cells. The principal active compound in artichokes is cynarin.

Artichoke helps prevent the accumulation of fats in the liver and arteries and is used in the treatment of atherosclerosis and arteriosclerosis. In a controlled trial published in *Drug Research*, two groups of thirty patients with hyperlipidemia (elevated blood fat levels) were treated for fifty days with cynarin (500 mg) or a placebo. Cynarin produced a significant reduction in blood cholesterol levels, lipoprotein levels, and body weight. Artichoke is also effective in preventing elevated cholesterol when toxins such as alcohol are present. As a bile stimulant, artichoke can also help prevent gallstones and liver damage from environmental toxins.

Cynarin decreases the rate of cholesterol synthesis in the liver and increases its conversion into bile acids. It also facilitates the flow of bile from the gallbladder and increases the contractive power of the bile ducts. In studies, artichoke has been shown to increase the production and volume of bile flow by as much as four times in a twelve-hour period. Artichokes also interrupt the enterohepatic circuit that would otherwise recirculate toxins between the gastrointestinal tract and the liver. Finally, artichokes stimulate the regeneration of liver cells.

Suggested Dosage: Artichoke is generally recognized as safe by the FDA. Persons who are experiencing an acute episode of pain and spasm due to inflammation of the gallbladder should not take artichoke as it may aggravate the symptoms. Artichoke is available in 160 mg capsules; take one to two capsules three times per day.

Turmeric

Turmeric is an indispensable part of the mixture of spices known as curry powder. Curcumin is the medicinally active compound in turmeric; the rich orange-yellow pigment that gives turmeric its characteristic color. Turmeric has been used for thousands of years in Indian cooking and in India's traditional Ayurvedic medicine. The turmeric plant, grown from India to Indonesia, is related to ginger and has pulpy, orange, tuberous roots that grow to about two feet in length.

Turmeric is widely used in indigenous medicine in the treatment of jaundice and liver disease. Herbalists prescribe it to prevent liver damage from alcohol and other toxins. Turmeric is also known to promote circulation, dissolve blood clots, and treat irregular menstruation of all kinds.

In India it is applied topically to treat fresh wounds, bruises, and insect bites. Animal studies have shown curcumin to be an effective treatment for acute and chronic inflammation, and curcumin is used in the, acute and chronic inflammation of the gallbladder, treatment of gallstones, and inflammation of the bile duct.

In a study in *The Journal of Nutrition*, curcumin lowered serum and liver cholesterol by one-half to one-third. Turmeric is also used as a digestive aid, facilitating the digestion of fats, hence its medicinal usefulness in curry.

Curcumin increases bile secretion and the contraction of the gallbladder, thereby facilitating detoxification and potentially lowering cholesterol. Curcumin also functions as an anti-inflammatory and anticoagulant agent. It has been shown to increase levels of glutathione-S-transferase and UDP glucuronyl transferase, two liver enzymes important for the promotion of phase II detoxification reactions. In addition, curcumin has been shown to have an antibacterial action and to block tumor growth.

Suggested Dosage: Turmeric is on the FDA's list of herbs generally regarded as safe. However, because turmeric has a potential anticlotting effect, anyone with a blood-clotting problem or who is currently taking anticoagulant medications should consult with their physician before taking this herb. Turmeric should not be taken by pregnant or nursing women. Turmeric is available in 400 or 500 mg capsules; take one capsule two to three times per day.

Licorice root

The use of licorice has a long history, appearing prominently in the first great Chinese herbal The Pen Tsao Ching (Classic of Herbs), written more than 5000 years ago. Licorice today is one of the most prescribed herbs in the Chinese pharmacopoeia, second only to ginseng. Licorice has also long been used in the West for medicinal purposes. Bundles of licorice were found amid the treasures of King Tut's tomb, and licorice appears in European herbals (an herbal is a book about plants) from the Renaissance to modern times, usually prescribed and referenced as a diuretic.

The primary active component in licorice is glycyrrhizin, which has a broad range of benefits. The licorice root is fifty times sweeter than sugar. In studies, licorice has been used effectively to control hepatitis and improve liver function in people with cirrhosis.

Contemporary herbalists recommend licorice for its soothing effects on the respiratory and gastrointestinal tracts. In a study published in *The Lancet*, fifty patients with gastric ulcers were successfully treated with licorice, which was as effective as treatment with a drug such as cimetidine. Licorice also has important anti-inflammatory properties. It stimulates cell production of interferon, the body's own antiviral compound. Licorice can also be used in nutritional programs to treat bacterial and fungal infections.

Suggested Dosage: Licorice is included in the FDA's list of herbs generally regarded as safe. Overdose reports have involved highly concentrated licorice extracts used in some candies, laxatives, and tobacco products. There have been no reports of problems caused by licorice sticks or the powdered herb.

However, licorice should not be used by pregnant and nursing women or by anyone with a history of diabetes, glaucoma, high blood pressure, stroke, or heart disease, as licorice can cause water retention and a rise in blood pressure.

To take licorice as a tea, gently boil and then simmer ½ tsp. of the powdered herb in one cup of water for ten minutes. Drink up to two cups a day. Licorice root is also available in 300 mg capsules; take one capsule between meals two times per day.

A Caution on the Use of Herbs

The use of herbs in individuals with impaired detoxification capabilities can be a double-edged sword: Certain herbs have very powerful liver-cleansing and restorative effects. However, sensitive individuals may not be able to process these herbs, which then overwhelm the very detoxification system that needs to be strengthened. These individuals may have immediate unpleasant side effects such as nausea, abdominal bloating, and congestion, and discomfort in the region of the liver. Such individuals should avoid the use of liver-cleansing herbs entirely until their detoxification capability is greatly strengthened. If you want to try an herbal program and are unsure of your tolerance for herbs, start with one-quarter of the suggested dosages. If this is well tolerated, you can gradually increase your intake over several weeks to therapeutic levels.

Green Foods

Green foods are important ingredients in herbal cleansing programs because chlorophyll, that imparts the green color to these foods, helps to neutralize and remove toxins. The greener the plant, the greater the amount of chlorophyll. Foods high in chlorophyll also help heal digestive disorders, provide energy, boost immunity, and prevent deficiency diseases such as anemia. Certain grasses and algae, which are described below, are especially high in chlorophyll.

As cited in an article published in *Mutation Research,* the National Institute for Occupational Safety and Health estimated that millions of workers in the manufacturing field have been exposed to potentially hazardous chemicals, many of which cause genetic mutation and promote cancer.

This same article reports on a study that shows the effectiveness of chlorophyll in counteracting the mutagenic effect of pollutants such as diesel-emission particles coal dust and cigarette smoke. Chlorophyll was extremely effective at inhibiting the mutations of the various nitrogen compounds, aromatic amines, and hydrocarbons found in these substances. Chlorophyll also protected against harmful compounds in fried beef and pork, red grape juice, and red wine. Chlorophyll has also been used successfully to treat iron deficiency anemia when used with iron supplements and peptic ulcers.

Pure extracted liquid chlorophyll is available in health food stores. Always use chlorophyll that has been extracted from alfalfa or other plants; avoid the chemically manufactured variety. There is a benefit to consuming the plant itself as a source of chlorophyll, since grasses and algae offer their own additional properties.

Suggested Dosage: 100 mg two or three times a day.

Wheat grass and barley grass

Cereal grasses, such as wheat grass and barley grass, are high-chlorophyll foods. Commercially, they are available fresh and as supplements, in both powder and tablet form. It is also possible to grow wheat grass at home. Both have nearly identical therapeutic properties, although barley grass may be digested a little more easily by some. People with allergies to wheat and other cereals can usually tolerate these grasses since grain in its grass stage rarely triggers an allergic reaction.

These grasses contain about the same quotient of protein as meat, about 20 percent, as well as vitamin B12, chlorophyll, vitamin A, and several other nutrients. Wheat grass is capable of incorporating more than 90 out of the estimated possible 102 minerals found in rich soil.

Wheat and barley grasses have been used to treat hepatitis and high cholesterol, as well as arthritis, peptic ulcers, and hypoglycemia. They are both effective in reducing inflammation and contain the antioxidant superoxide dismutase (SOD), which slows cellular deterioration, plus various digestive enzymes that aid in detoxification.

Suggested Dosage: Combine 1-2 tbsp. of the powder or 1 to 2 oz. of the fresh juice in 8 oz. of water.

Microalgae

Spirulina, chlorella, and wild blue-green algae contain more chlorophyll than any other foods. These algae are aquatic plants, spiral-shaped, emerald to blue-green in color, and have been used medicinally for thousands of years in South America and Africa. Today they can be purchased, as a powder in health food stores.

They are also the highest sources of protein, beta-carotene, and nucleic acids of any animal or plant food, as well as containing the essential fatty acids omega-3 and gamma linolenic acid. The protein in spirulina and chlorella is so easily digested and absorbed that two or three teaspoons of these microalgae are equivalent to two to three ounces of meat. Further, unlike animal protein, the protein in algae generates a minimum of waste products when it is metabolized, thereby lessening stress on the liver.

Spirulina. Spirulina detoxifies the kidneys and liver, inhibiting the growth of fungi, bacteria, and yeasts. Because spirulina is so easily digested, it yields quick energy. It is also strongly anti-inflammatory and therefore useful in the treatment of hepatitis, gastritis, and other inflammatory diseases. Spirulina strengthens body tissues and protects the vascular system by lowering blood fat. Athletes use spirulina for energy and for its cleansing action after strenuous physical exertion, which can stimulate the body to rid itself of poisons.

Suggested Dosage: A standard dosage of spirulina is 1 to 2 tbsp stirred into 8 oz. of water per day. Green foods are very concentrated, so start with a half dose and increase gradually to ensure it is well tolerated.

Chlorella. This well-known algae is an especially effective detoxifier and anti-inflammatory agent because it is high in chlorophyll, which stimulates these processes. Chlorella is notable for its tough outer cell walls, which bind with heavy metals, pesticides, and carcinogens such as PCBs (polychlorinated biphenyls) and then carry these toxins out of the body. Because of chlorella's growth factor, this algae also promotes growth and repair of all kinds of tissue. Animal studies show that it reduces cholesterol and atherosclerosis.

Suggested Dosage: 1 tbsp. taken in 8 to 12 oz. of water. Green foods are very concentrated. Be sure to begin with a partial dose and increase gradually.

Wild blue-green algae. Wild blue-green algae grows in Klamath Lake in Oregon and is processed by freeze-drying. It is sold under various trade names, frequently as a mail-order product. Wild blue-green algae is very energizing and can improve an individual's mental concentration. However, a sign of over use is weakness and a lack of mental focus, and certain forms are known to be highly toxic.

Many of my female patients who are in their late thirties and forties report that taking blue-green algae helps lessen the fatigue and mood swings associated with PMS and perimenopausal hormone imbalances. While I have not found it to be helpful in reducing physical symptoms such as bloating, breast tenderness, and menstrual irregularity, it does seem to promote more efficient liver function. Since the liver has a crucial role in detoxifying and deactivating estrogen, healthy liver function helps to bring estrogen levels into balance, thereby relieving the depression fatigue and moodiness often found in perimenopausal women.

Suggested Dosage: 1 tbsp. daily in 8 to 12 oz. of water. It is important to buy wild blue-green algae from a reputable company that processes the algae in an FDA-approved laboratory. To avoid certain wild blue-green algae that is highly toxic, never collect it yourself or consume any that you have gathered.

Various green foods can be combined in an easy-to-digest, highly nutritious drink. As with all concentrated foods, begin with small amounts and work up to your final level. In my personal recipe, I use 1 tbsp of a wheat and barley grass combination and 2 tbsp of spirulina. Add water to a consistency you enjoy, and combine using either a whisk or a blender. If you use a blender, be sure to empty the container and then add back some additional water to remove all the green foods, as they are expensive and you do not want to waste them.

13

Liver-Cleansing Techniques

Liver flushes and coffee enemas are very effective detoxification techniques that directly stimulate the liver and gallbladder to release accumulated poisons. They are best used as part of an overall detoxification program that incorporates adequate water, exercise, a modified diet, nutritional supplements, and rest. I discuss how to use these techniques in this chapter.

Because a rigorous detoxification program can be extremely disruptive to a person's life, I recommend a slower, gentler, more gradual process of detoxification accomplished with a lighter diet (as outlined in chapter 8), which will cause fewer side effects.

When it comes to detoxification, intense is not always better. A rigorous cleanse is more appropriate for times of relaxation and retreat when a person has the available time to take saunas, lounge in the sun, and read books. However, if you want to take a more aggressive approach, you may want to experiment with the following cleanses, which accelerate detoxification. These include a coffee enema, liver flush, colon cleansing, sauna, and dry brush massage.

Using Coffee for a Powerful Detoxification Technique

Although the procedure may sound unusual, coffee enemas have been used as a detoxification technique for at least 100 years. As cited in *The Townsend Letter for Doctors & Patients*, animal studies conducted in Germany in the 1920s found that a caffeine solution administered rectally tends to stimulate the production of bile.

Max Gerson, M.D., a pioneer in liver detoxification techniques, incorporated coffee enemas into his now well-known cancer protocol. He recommended that a regimen of coffee enemas be strictly followed, both in the clinic and at home, for at least 18 months. The noted New York immunologist Nicholas Gonzalez, M.D. also includes coffee enemas as part of an overall program to treat cancer. According to Dr. Gonzalez, the enemas facilitate elimination of the waste products and toxins that can accumulate as tumors break down.

Coffee enemas flood only the sigmoid, or lower, portion of the bowel. When coffee is taken into the lower bowel, nearly all of the caffeine in it is absorbed, first into the hemorrhoidal veins, then into the portal veins, and eventually into the liver.

The caffeine causes these blood vessels and the liver's bile ducts to dilate (expand), thereby increasing the release of bile. The fluid in the bowel dilutes the bile, triggering a further increase in bile flow. In addition, a coffee enema significantly increases glutathione S-transferase levels, an enzyme that catalyzes the release of bile.

A coffee enema that lasts ten to twelve minutes can facilitate significant purging of toxins from the liver and colon. In addition, caffeine causes smooth muscle in the liver and gallbladder to relax, which can be therapeutic for individuals with spastic colon and irritable-bowel syndrome.

Ingredients and equipment

It is important to use coffee that is both caffeinated and organic. Using nonorganic coffee beans, most of which are sprayed with pesticides, would undermine the purpose of the technique, which is to purge the body of toxins. When making the coffee, use water that is free of chlorine and fluorides. The water can be distilled, filtered, or spring water from a glass container (water stored in a plastic container may contain toxic chemicals that leached into it from the plastic).

Procedure

The actual procedure for a coffee enema is relatively simple and can become routine.

First, make the coffee. Use three rounded tablespoons of organic drip ground caffeinated coffee to one quart of pure water. Boil the coffee for five minutes, then lower the heat and simmer it for fifteen to twenty minutes. Strain the coffee and cool it to body temperature.

Next, lay a towel on the floor. Put the enema bag in the sink with the catheter closed, and pour 8 to 16 ounces of the prepared coffee into the bag. Loosen the catheter clamp to allow the coffee to flow to the tip of the catheter, and reclamp it when all the air is removed from the tubing. Then hang the filled bag from a door handle or towel rack near where you are going to lie down to generate a gentle flow of liquid.

Lie down on the towel on the floor and insert catheter into the rectum a few inches, using a lubricant if needed. Lie on your right side in a fetal position, with both thighs drawn close to the abdomen. Release the clamp and slowly let the coffee flow into the colon. Breathe deeply. If you experience any discomfort or fullness, immediately close the clamp.

Retain the fluid for ten minutes to insure that caffeine reaches the bile ducts of the liver. Feel free to change position to insure the greatest degree of comfort. When the time limit is reached, be sure to expel the enema completely as with normal elimination. If you have an immediate urge to release the coffee, do so to empty the colon of stool, then repeat the procedure. When you are done, rinse the enema bag thoroughly with soap and water and hang it to dry. You can also clean it using boiling water or hydrogen peroxide to prevent mold growth.

Cautions for coffee enemas

The complementary physicians who recommend this technique, report that coffee enemas can be taken once or even several times a day during the early stages of a detoxification program without toxic effects. There is no indication that enemas disrupt normal voiding; in fact, people often report less constipation. There is also little risk of flushing out vitamins and minerals because these are absorbed from the stool before it reaches the sigmoid portion of the bowel.

If symptoms of toxicity occur—such as headache, fever, nausea, intestinal spasms, and fatigue—take the enemas less frequently or stop their use entirely. Individuals with chronic diarrhea or inflammatory bowel disease should use this technique cautiously or not at all. If you have any questions about the advisability of using coffee enemas for your particular case, I recommend that you discuss this with your own health care provider.

Liver Flushes

A liver flush is a drink of fruit juice and olive oil, which increases the flow of bile from the liver, helps to eliminate toxins, and thereby assists in the restoration of liver function. For a gradual cleanse, liver flushes may be done several consecutive days. It is beneficial to consult an experienced complementary health care professional if you wish to do a series of these, since different practitioners may suggest various programs.

However, if you want to do a liver flush on an unsupervised basis, they may be done for a period of up to ten days. Since the flush is made up, partly, of low-pH citrus fruit juices, it should be used cautiously or avoided entirely by individuals who are overly acidic. This type of flush is best tolerated by individuals with healthy acid/alkaline balance and high alkaline producers. If you have any questions or concerns about the advisability of doing liver flushes in your particular case, I recommend that you discuss this with your own health care provider.

The following liver flush has a pleasing taste and can be made as follows:

1. Combine 6 oz. of an orange/grapefruit juice mixture with 2 oz. of either lime or lemon juice. This mixture will taste relatively acidic and astringent (it may make your mouth pucker). Traditionally, such mixtures are used to neutralize the deleterious effects of a high-fat, high-protein diet on the liver and help to promote liver cleansing.

2. Pour the juice mixture into a glass jar with a tight-fitting lid (or in a blender), and add one or two cloves of fresh squeezed garlic and ½ tsp. grated fresh ginger.

3. To this juice and herb mixture, add 1 tbsp. extra-virgin olive oil. Finally, dilute this mixture with up to 6 oz. of spring or filtered water. Close the lid securely and thoroughly shake the mixture to combine ingredients or blend in the blender.

4. Drink the liver flush slowly. It is best to take the flush early in the morning, apart from meals, and to follow it with an herbal tea such as peppermint or chamomile, both of which have a mildly cleansing effect on the liver.

Colon Cleanses

Colon cleanses are an important component of detox-ification. A colon cleanse removes toxins from the walls of the intestines, where they may have accumulated over time; it can also lessen the stress of toxins on the liver. Waste products are excreted either via the kidneys, intestines, or skin, but the majority of waste products leaving the liver pass from the body through the bowels. How efficiently and quickly the body can rid itself of these toxins directly depends on how well the colon is cleansed, which can speed transit time of conjugated chemicals and prevent their reabsorption into the body.

Fiber, dietary or supplemental, is a very effective colon cleanser. A diet that lacks fiber is usually high in fat, and this combination promotes the reabsorp-tion of cholesterol and hormones. In contrast, a high fiber diet binds both cholesterol and estrogen effectively, and enhances their elimination from the body from the intestinal tract. There are two main types of fiber, insoluble and soluble. In addition, clay products can have similar effects to those of fiber.

Insoluble fiber

Insoluble fiber is mostly indigestible cellulose, which makes up the skin of fruits and vegetables and the cover of cereal grains such as wheat germ. Eating an apple along with its skin or brown rice rather than white provides insoluble fiber. Other fibers include the hemicelluloses.

A good example is psyllium seed husks, which are an essential part of colon cleanses, binding the toxins released from the liver during detoxification. Psyllium is able to hold water, thereby softening and moisturizing the intestinal tract as it passes through the bowel. And because psyllium is similar to the mucosa of the intestines, it is able to keep debris from sticking to the walls of the intestines. Sometimes psyllium treatment is accompanied by the use of an herbal laxative such as senna, which speeds the elimination of bound toxins. I usually recommend 1 to 2 tbsp. of psyllium stirred into 12 to 16 oz. of water. You should drink this immediately, as psyllium will tend to form a gel.

Soluble fiber

Guar gum is a soluble fiber that is extracted from the guar plant, grown in the Middle East. It is included in detoxification protocols as an intestinal binder and laxative. It easily absorbs cold water, forming a thick, pastelike substance (the reason it is often an ingredient in commercial ice cream and cheese spreads). As a dietary fiber, it also assists the liver in managing cholesterol levels, lowering LDL cholesterol (which is associated with a higher risk of heart disease), increasing bile secretion, and reducing the absorption of cholesterol. Stir ½ tsp. of guar gum into 8 to 12 oz. of water and drink immediately.

Pectin is another soluble fiber, found in most plants and particularly in fruits and vegetables such as apples and citrus. Pectin has a neutral, nonassertive flavor and is used as a food stabilizer and thickener. It is also a binding agent, prescribed extensively in Russia for the removal of environmental toxins from the body. As a supplement for detoxification, use 1 tsp. in 8 to 12 oz. of water, mix well, and drink immediately, before it jells. This drink can be taken twice a day. Guar gum and pectin can be combined. Pectin is also available in 500 mg capsules; take three capsules, one to three times per day.

Clays

Some holistic health care practitioners use clay products in a detoxification regimen. Bentonite is a powdered clay composed of minute particles that give the clay a very large surface area in proportion to its volume, allowing it to collect as much as forty times its weight in toxins. Liquid or hydrated Bentonite is most frequently used for internal detoxification, but any powdered clay can be added to water and soaked overnight for use the next day. Bentonite is available in premeasured regimens in natural-food stores.

A fiber success story

One of my patients, Adrienne, a forty-five-year-old financial consultant, had great success using fiber to improve her health. She had a busy and demanding business, with little time to eat lunch. She would often eat a quick meal consisting of a burger or tacos at one of the surrounding fast-food restaurants near her office.

She came to me complaining of constipation, with bowel movements only every three or four days, bloating, morning brain fog—symptoms typical of toxicity and poor elimination. She was 20 pounds overweight, and her cholesterol was quite elevated, a particular concern since she had a strong family history of heart disease.

With my counsel, Adrienne slowly improved her overall diet, and she began to take bag lunches with her to work, which included raw vegetables like carrots and celery, and whole grain breads for fiber. If she ate a burrito or taco, it was homemade with brown rice, beans, and with no added fat.

Adrienne began to take a daily fiber-rich drink made with 1 tsp. guar gum and 1 tsp. pectin dissolved in 12 oz. of water. In addition, she took 2 tbsp. of psyllium mixed with water every day. When she came back to my office for a three-month checkup, Adrienne reported having bowel movements once or twice a day; she had lost fifteen pounds and her cholesterol had dropped significantly. She was very pleased with the results and totally committed to continuing the program.

Maintaining intestinal flora

A colon cleanse can remove healthy flora from the intestines, so it is important to reintroduce friendly, live bacteria into the intestines after a detoxification program is completed to maintain proper digestion. Yogurt and other fermented foods such as kefir contain the beneficial bacteria Lactobacillus acidophilus.

Prebiotics, a therapy developed in Japan, is designed to feed the beneficial bacteria. Fructooligosaccharides (FOSs) are naturally occurring carbohydrates that promote the growth of the healthful bacteria Bifidobacteria and lactobacilli. As a supplement, FOS comes in dry powder form and as a syrup. FOS is readily available in natural-food stores. Follow the directions listed on the packaging of the product you buy. These carbohydrates are also found in honey, garlic, asparagus, tomato, onions, banana, rye, barley, and triticale.

Therapeutic Baths, Sweats, and Saunas

The skin is the largest organ of elimination in the body. Besides excreting essential minerals when we perspire, the skin is also a route for the excretion of waste products. Any detoxification program must include regular bathing and, can be enhanced by activities that accelerate sweating, such as saunas and exercise.

Many people are aware that spending some time in a hot tub or sauna hydrates and relaxes the body, but few think of the health benefits in terms of detoxification. Relaxing in this way also benefits the internal organs of elimination, the liver and kidneys, by lessening the amount of toxins they must process.

When taking sweats and saunas, be sure to drink ample water, and supplement your diet with potassium, calcium, and magnesium to replace the minerals lost in perspiration. Combinations of these nutrients are available in natural-food stores. Also, avoid becoming overheated.

Some people take niacin, which causes flushing and additional perspiring. To avoid an exaggerated niacin flush, which can be stressful, begin by supplementing with only 10 to 50 mg daily, gradually increasing to a maximum dose of 100 mg per day.

A Home-Spa Cleansing Treatment

When you have some leisure time to yourself, plan a few days of juice fasting, thirty minutes to an hour of regular aerobic exercise, and a daily sauna or hot tub. Such days of renewal are best spent quietly in contemplation or meditation. Most people find that they feel greatly refreshed after spending even a few days doing such a program.

Dry Brush Massages

You can easily incorporate dry brush massage into a program of cleansing, adding it to your normal daily routine of washing. Dry brushing removes dead surface skin and increases superficial circulation throughout the body. Many alternative healers use dry brush massage to facilitate detoxification, on the theory that it stimulates the lymphatic system. The lymphatic system is the network of ducts or channels that transport lymph, the clear fluid that accumulates in the spaces between cells and in the capillaries. Like the circulatory system, the lymphatic system helps to move fluid through the body and carries toxins to the liver for breakdown and excretion.

To give yourself a dry brush massage, use a moderately soft, natural vegetable-fiber bristle brush, and rub the skin vigorously to stimulate it and remove dead cells. Then brush your body, front, back, and limbs, using light but brisk short strokes. Start at the extremities and stroke in the direction of your navel, moving from the wrists to the armpits, the chin to the navel, and the feet up to the groin. Brush gently at first, as some parts of the body may be especially sensitive.

The massage should take no more than ten minutes daily. As your body becomes accustomed to the massage, this routine can be done daily for three months, and then twice a week as part of a preventive maintenance program. Putting sea salt on the brush will cause the pores of the skin to open further for an even more cleansing effect.

Sea Salt and Soda Baths

I particularly love sea salt and soda baths because they are a relaxing and gentle way to detoxify the body and can be enjoyed several times a week. These baths are alkaline and are deeply restorative to the body by promoting a healthy acid/alkaline balance.

A healthy acid/alkaline balance is beneficial for your energy, balanced mood, immunity, healthy bones, heart and kidney health and many other essential functions.

Fill a bathtub with warm water and add one cup of baking soda (sodium bicarbonate) plus one cup of sea salt or one pound of Epsom salt. You can also add therapeutic essential oils like lavender or rose water for their relaxation benefits and beautiful scents.

Stay in the bath for twenty to thirty minutes to have the full detoxification benefits.

Ginger Baths

Would you like to detox your body and feel refreshed, full of energy and vitality? Ginger baths are a great way to receive these benefits!

To do a ginger bath, fill your tub with warm water. Add 2 cups of Epsom salts to your tub. Epsom salts are magnesium sulfate which you will absorb through the water. They relax your muscles, joints, reduce stiffness and tension and even flush out toxins. In addition, add 1 to 2 cups of baking soda which will make your bath more alkaline to help balance your pH and leave your skin feeling soft and smooth.

Finally, add 1 tablespoon to 1/4 cup of ground ginger to your tub. I recommend adding the ginger slowly to the tub to your tolerance level since it will cause your skin to slightly flush and will help you to sweat out toxins.

Ginger can cause much sweating and detoxification so make sure that you do it to a level that feels comfortable and isn't too intense. Try to stay in the tub from 20 to 40 minutes or to your level of comfort if you need to stay in for shorter periods of time.

After getting out of the bath, I recommend that you wrap yourself in a large towel or blanket since you will continue to detoxify through sweating for the next few hours.

Get out of the bathtub slowly since you may feel lightheaded and tired initially from the detoxification. Be sure to drink plenty of water to help flush out toxins and replace any fluid loss. Taking a multivitamin/mineral supplement can help to further replenish any nutrients.

Regular Exercise

Aerobic exercise such as walking helps the body to detoxify since circulation is enhanced and toxins are more efficiently excreted through the urinary tract, bowels, and skin. Exercise increases metabolic rate and tones the liver so that it can metabolize fats better, as well as burning calories. If you are consuming potentially toxic substances such as alcohol and sugar, regular aerobic exercise is essential and should be done, most beneficially, nearly every day or at least every other day for thirty minutes to one hour.

During an aerobic workout, the heartbeat should remain elevated for at least thirty minutes. After exercising, be sure to shower to wash away the toxins excreted in perspiration, which may be reabsorbed if they remain on the skin.

Oxygen Therapies

Oxygen therapies can increase oxygenation and circulation through the liver, thereby enhancing the detoxification process. They can be tremendously useful in restoring liver function and are used in treating liver diseases such as hepatitis. Oxygen therapies are discussed in detail in my book on this topic.

Summary of Treatment Options for Restoring Your Ability to Detoxify

Diet
- o The detoxification diet
- o Modified fasting

Nutrients to restore liver function
- o Lecithin
- o Amino acids
  - Methionine
  - Glutathione
  - Cysteine
  - N-acetyl cysteine (NAC)
- o Essential fatty acids
- o Herbs
  - Milk thistle plant (silymarin)
  - Dandelion
  - Artichoke
  - Curcumin (turmeric)
  - Licorice root
- o Green foods
  - Wheat grass and barley grass
  - Microalgae

Liver-cleansing techniques
- o Coffee enema
- o Fiber intake
- o Maintaining intestinal flora
- o Dry brush massage
- o Sea salt and soda baths
- o Ginger baths
- o Regular aerobic exercise
- o Oxygen therapies

About Susan Richards, M.D.

Dr. Susan Richards is one of the foremost authorities in the fields of family medicine and alternative medicine. Dr. Richards has successfully treated many thousands of patients emphasizing alternative health and integrative medicine in her clinical practice. Her mission is to provide her patients with safe and effective alternative therapies to greatly enhance their health and well-being.

A graduate of Northwestern University Feinberg School of Medicine, she has served on the clinical faculty of Stanford University School of Medicine and taught in their Division of Family and Community Medicine.

Her Facebook page, Dr. Susan's Healthy Living, has over one million followers. She is also an ordained minister and her ministry receives over a million prayer requests for healing each year.

Notes

Notes

www.ingramcontent.com/pod-product-compliance
Lightning Source LLC
Chambersburg PA
CBHW070903290526
45795CB00001B/217